MAYO CLINIC

GUIDE TO

BETTER SLEEP

Find relief from insomnia,
sleep apnea, and other sleep disorders

 Press

MAYO CLINIC PRESS

Medical Editors | Timothy I. Morgenthaler, M.D.; Bhanu Prakash Kolla, M.B.B.S., M.D.
Contributors | Mithri Junna, M.D.; Melissa C. Lipford, M.D.
Writer | Peter Kendall
Publisher | Daniel J. Harke
Editor in Chief | Nina E. Wiener
Senior Editor | Karen R. Wallevand
Art Director | Stewart J. Koski
Production Design | Darren L. Wendt
Illustration and Photography | Mayo Clinic Media Support Services, Mayo Clinic Medical Illustration and Animation
Editorial Research Librarians | Eddy S. Morrow, Jr.; Erika A. Riggin
Image Credits | All photographs and illustrations are copyright of Mayo Foundation for Medical Education and Research (MFMER) except for the following: Cover (front and back), CREDIT: filo/DigitalVision Vectors/Getty Images; maaikeart/500px/500Px Plus

When you purchase Mayo Clinic newsletters and books, proceeds are used to further medical education and research at Mayo Clinic.

Copyright © 2025 Mayo Foundation for Medical Education and Research (MFMER)

MAYO, MAYO CLINIC and the Mayo triple-shield logo are marks of Mayo Foundation for Medical Education and Research. All rights reserved. No part of this book may be reproduced, stored in a retrieval system, or transmitted, in any form or by any means, electronic, mechanical, photocopying, recording or otherwise, without the prior written permission of the publisher.

The information in this book is true and complete to the best of our knowledge. This book is intended only as an informative guide for those wishing to learn more about health issues. It is not intended to replace, countermand or conflict with advice given to you by your own physician. The ultimate decision concerning your care should be made between you and your doctor. Information in this book is offered with no guarantees. The author and publisher disclaim all liability in connection with the use of this book.

For bulk sales to employers, member groups and health-related companies, email SpecialSalesMayoBooks@mayo.edu. To stay informed about Mayo Clinic Press, please subscribe to our free e-newsletter at MCPress.MayoClinic.org or follow us on social media.

ISBN: 979-8-88770-049-6 (hardcover)
ISBN: 979-8-88770-050-2 (ebook)

Library of Congress Control Number: 2024013109

Library of Congress Cataloging-in-Publication Data

Names: Morgenthaler, Timothy I., author. | Kolla, Bhanu Prakash (Professor of Psychiatry), author.

Title: Mayo clinic guide to better sleep : find relief from insomnia, sleep apnea and other sleep disorders / Timothy I. Morgenthaler, Bhanu Prakash Kolla.

Description: Rochester, MN : Mayo Clinic Press, [2025] | Includes index. |

Identifiers: LCCN 2024013109 | ISBN 9798887700496 (hardcover) | ISBN 9798887700502 (ebook)

Subjects: LCSH: Sleep — Health aspects. | Sleep disorders.

Classification: LCC RA786 .M327 2025 | DDC 613.7/94 — dc23/eng/20240523

LC record available at https://lccn.loc.gov/2024013109

Printed in the United States

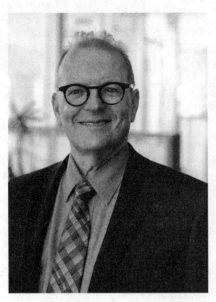 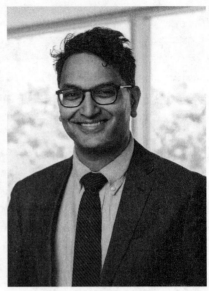

Timothy I. Morgenthaler, M.D., is a sleep medicine specialist and the director of Mayo Clinic's Center for Sleep Medicine in Rochester, Minnesota. A professor of medicine in the Mayo Clinic College of Medicine and Science, he also serves as a vice chair for quality at Mayo Clinic, and as the associate chair for innovation in the Division of Pulmonary and Critical Care Medicine. Dr. Morgenthaler's clinical practice focuses on the treatment of patients with central and obstructive sleep apnea, sleep-related breathing disorders and other adult sleep disorders. His research interests include outcomes research, novel techniques, device innovation and healthcare delivery in the areas of sleep medicine, earning him the Nathaniel Kleitman Distinguished Service Award from the American Academy of Sleep Medicine, where he is a fellow.

Bhanu Prakash Kolla, M.B.B.S., M.D., is a professor of psychiatry and psychology at Mayo Clinic College of Medicine and Science, Rochester, Minnesota. A psychiatrist with specialty training in sleep medicine and addiction psychiatry, Dr. Kolla is an expert in the overlap between sleep disorders and addiction. He practices at Mayo Clinic's Center for Sleep Medicine and in the Division of Addiction Medicine. Dr. Kolla's research interests include management of sleep disruptions associated with alcohol and substance abuse recovery, and the management of treatment-resistant insomnia. He is a fellow of the American Psychiatric Association, the American Academy of Sleep Medicine and the Royal College of Psychiatry, and a frequent speaker at national and international conferences.

Table of contents

7	From the editors
11	**CHAPTER 1:** **UNDERSTANDING SLEEP**
35	**CHAPTER 2:** **HOW MUCH SLEEP DO YOU NEED?**
53	**CHAPTER 3:** **WHEN SLEEP IS INTERRUPTED**
81	**CHAPTER 4:** **IN SEARCH OF QUALITY SLEEP**
105	**CHAPTER 5:** **DO YOU HAVE A SLEEP DISORDER?**
124	**CHAPTER 6:** **INSOMNIA**
153	**CHAPTER 7:** **SLEEP MEDICATIONS**

175	**CHAPTER 8:**
	SLEEP APNEA

206	**CHAPTER 9:**
	TREATING SLEEP APNEA

230	**CHAPTER 10:**
	NARCOLEPSY AND IDIOPATHIC INSOMNIA

245	**CHAPTER 11:**
	RESTLESS LEGS SYNDROME

264	**CHAPTER 12:**
	UNUSUAL BEHAVIORS DURING SLEEP

282	**CHAPTER 13:**
	INTERNAL SLEEP-CLOCK DISORDERS

295	**CHAPTER 14:**
	MEDICAL CONDITIONS AND MEDICATIONS

307	Final thoughts
309	Additional resources
311	Index

From the editors

Most people who write a book don't set out to put you to sleep. But we understand better than almost anyone how difficult it is for many people to get quality sleep, and we know that we can help.

The two of us have been practicing sleep medicine for more than 50 years combined, and we have the honor and privilege of working at Mayo Clinic's Center for Sleep Medicine, a pioneering sleep clinic at one of the finest medical centers in the world. We wrote this book to share what we and other experts in our field have learned in recent decades, because we know that improving sleep can be life-changing. And to be honest, we both also love sleep medicine and can't resist sharing some of the truly amazing discoveries about why we need sleep, how we sleep and the many ways that sleep can run amok.

First, we'd like to tell you a little about who we are and how we became sleep specialists. Sleep is so central to mental and physical health that it brought the two of us to the same field, even though we got there through very different interests and medical disciplines.

Dr. Morgenthaler
After my training in the U.S. Navy in surgery and undersea and diving medicine, I came to Mayo Clinic, where I received additional education and began my career as a pulmonologist, a doctor who treats breathing conditions. I was drawn to the relationship between breathing and sleep and how the two are intertwined in elegant and complex ways. I also saw how many people are affected by sleep-related breathing disorders. It didn't take long for me to fall in love with sleep medicine.

One case early in my career dramatically demonstrated to me how disturbed sleep can lead to other, seemingly unrelated health problems, with a profound impact on a person's well-being.

I was approached by a psychiatrist caring for a middle-aged man in the psychiatric unit. The poor fellow had developed psychosis, and doctors couldn't understand how he got that way. More importantly, efforts to treat him were severely hampered by the fact that it seemed he couldn't sleep. The patient wasn't able to speak coherently or participate in therapy.

During a difficult interview, I was able to determine that for many years this man had suffered from what I thought quite likely was restless legs syndrome, a disorder you can read about in this book. I immediately prescribed treatment for the condition and within two nights the man was sleeping 4 to 6 hours at a time. His symptoms rapidly improved and some months later it was determined that he didn't have a severe psychiatric condition after all. Rather, his problem was sleep deprivation as a result of his restless legs disorder.

As my patient load grew and I saw how many people's lives were changed with improved sleep, I became convinced that I wanted to invest more of my time and energy into the practice, research, and education of sleep medicine. It's what I enjoy today at Mayo Clinic.

Dr. Kolla
My career path was shaped by two diverse cultural and medical landscapes — medical school in the vibrant heart of India and the scholarly ambience of the United Kingdom's Oxford Deanery, where I completed a psychiatry residency.

My fascination with the human mind and its complexities led me to explore the intricate interplay between mental health and substance use disorders. During my encounters with patients, I learned that sleep also was a fundamental influence. And it became increasingly apparent that to treat my patients, I had to understand the nighttime aspects of their lives to improve their daytime functioning. This led me to the field of sleep medicine and to Mayo Clinic, where I received additional training.

One case I remember well took place during my residency and involved a man being treated for alcohol addiction. He described significant difficulties with falling and staying asleep, a problem that spanned more than seven years. Because of his insomnia, he suffered from fatigue, loss of concentration and an inability to perform his job as a teacher.

The patient discovered that having a nightcap could help him fall asleep. However, very quickly he developed a tolerance to alcohol. He started drinking more, but soon realized that it was no longer helping him sleep. After his withdrawal symptoms were treated, the man was still plagued by ongoing sleep difficulties and worried about a relapse to alcohol. With the use of behavioral strategies and a short-term sleeping pill, I helped him allay his anxieties so that he could complete treatment and be successful in his recovery.

From this encounter, it became clear to me that a substantial proportion of the patients in my psychiatry practice had significant sleep problems, and treating their sleep disturbances could have a profound impact on their mental health and overall well-being. Today my research and clinical practice reflect a comprehensive approach that encompasses the intersection of sleep, addiction and psychiatry.

How this book can help you

Although we came to sleep medicine via these two very different paths — pulmonology and psychiatry — our experiences in the field have led us to a shared understanding of how to approach sleep problems while caring for the whole person. A small but important aspect of this approach is our belief that the more someone understands sleep and the many ways that it can be disturbed, the better equipped they are to improve it.

In this book, we explain the fundamentals of sleep science at some length. While we don't shy away from the science, we present the information in a clear and simplified approach, making it easy for you to understand. Discoveries in the last few decades have changed our understanding of sleep and its effect on the brain and body. This information has great practical value for anyone trying to understand their own sleep troubles, or those of a loved one, and how to address them. (Of course, the two of us find the science of sleep fascinating and thrilling in its own right!)

The information in the pages that follow stems from our experiences in helping thousands of people searching for better sleep as well as the latest published research and the advice of professional medical associations. It can serve as both a starting place and an ongoing reference for anyone who wants to sleep better.

Understanding that someone who believes they have a specific disorder, such as insomnia, for example, might be most interested in the chapter that focuses specifically on that condition, our goal was for certain chapters to be as complete and self-contained as possible. But other chapters, especially those early in the book, also include interesting and helpful information. So, we encourage you to check out the entire book.

We want to stress that this book isn't intended to equip you to diagnose and treat sleep disorders on your own. Only a physician can diagnose a sleep condition, and often a certified sleep specialist may be best suited to do so. However, we understand that not everyone has access to a sleep clinic and the deep expertise you can find there. The goal of the book is to help you understand your sleep and how it affects your health and well-being. This can make you a more informed partner as you and your physician work together to improve your sleep.

So, can *Mayo Clinic Guide to Better Sleep* really put you to sleep? Well, we certainly hope it's far too interesting to make you nod off while reading it. But we truly believe that the chapters here can help you on your journey to getting a better night's sleep and to gaining the many health benefits that come from that.

1

Understanding sleep

As a nation, we have a sleep problem. Constant pressures to stay connected, work harder and do more, while still fitting in some fun, are leaving us less time for sleep. And when we finally do find time to rest, we aren't sleeping well.

Everybody needs sleep, but healthy sleep — the kind that leaves you feeling alert and refreshed in the morning — is becoming more elusive. The numbers bear this out. More than one-third of Americans say they have difficulty sleeping, and a recent study placed the direct healthcare costs of the nation's sleep debt at nearly $100 billion annually.

Sleep is vital to good health. It can help keep your weight in check, keep your brain sharp and reduce your risk of common diseases such as heart disease, Alzheimer's, cancer and diabetes. Unfortunately, the tribulations and pressures of life, combined with unhealthy lifestyles and increased health concerns, are keeping many people from getting the sleep they need.

Whether you're desperately seeking a solution to your sleep woes or are simply curious if there's more you can do to improve your sleep and, ultimately, your health, the answer begins with understanding how sleep works and why it's so important.

YOUR BRAIN AT NIGHT

It's easy to think of sleep simply as a period of rest when your body shuts down and takes a break. Just the opposite: Sleep encompasses one of the most productive parts of your day — an astonishingly busy stretch when your body ticks through a lengthy to-do list to help keep you healthy and mentally sharp.

After a long day interacting with the world, during sleep your body turns its attention inward. It goes to work repairing cells, regrowing tissue and arming your immune system to hunt down invaders intent on causing disease or infection. At the same time, a cleaning system in your brain gives your cells a bath, washing away harmful waste products generated during a day of mental labor. Your brain sorts through the day's experiences, storing some as memories and tossing others as trivial and utterly forgettable. Acting something like its own therapist, your brain during sleep smooths out painful emotional edges and fortifies your resilience to face another day. Getting all this and more done each night is an elaborate production involving your brain's internal messaging systems, composed of hormones, chemical messengers and electrical impulses. You need sleep as much as you need food and water. Not just humans but every creature in the animal kingdom sleeps or has some kind of rest period.

Rather than a single long stretch of unconsciousness, sleep is made up of a number of distinct parts, each with its own purpose. As chemical messengers signal your body and your senses that it's time to shut out the outside world — to sleep — the brain's electrical activity slows in stages until it's nearly undetectable. But it doesn't remain that way the entire night. Occasionally it bursts to life again as if you were awake. This is because during sleep, your mind wanders dreamscapes of its own making, even causing your body to become virtually paralyzed at times.

While sleep can be a great pleasure, it also can be a terrible frustration. Your body and mind may conspire in many ways to keep you from getting the rest you so desperately need.

Sleep problems are common, at some point touching the lives of nearly everyone. Causes vary widely, ranging from the shape of your throat to the pressures and anxieties of modern life. Fortunately, most sleep conditions can be successfully managed or treated. Although you've been sleeping since before you were born, you can still learn new ways to improve your sleep; by doing so, you can reap countless benefits affecting how you think, feel and live, no matter your age.

In the remainder of this chapter, we walk you through how healthy sleep unfolds each night and the ways sleep is connected to nearly every part of your being — from how you feel to who you are. Understanding your sleeping brain will help you grasp why certain daily practices and behaviors can improve sleep and why others may be harmful, helping you to make informed decisions about what you can do to sleep and live better.

VITAL FUNCTIONS OF SLEEP

To some people, sleep can seem like a waste of time. Leonardo da Vinci and Thomas Edison famously tried to minimize the hours they spent asleep so they could accomplish more while awake. Perhaps this proves only that you can be a genius some of the time but not all the time. In fact, a good night's sleep boosts your ability to think clearly and creatively and improves your faculties for solving problems and remembering facts. It's not a stretch to say that sleep makes you smarter. (Albert Einstein, by the way, was an enthusiastic sleeper.)

From the deepest recesses of your brain to the skin at the tips of your fingers, every part of your body needs sleep. The list of vital functions carried out during sleep is long, influencing your entire well-being.

These tasks are orchestrated in part by two important processes affecting sleep: your body's daily patterns (circadian rhythms) and homeostasis. Circadian rhythms synchronize sleep and wakefulness with night and day. Unlike many animal species, which evolved to take advantage of being awake during darkness, humans took the diurnal path. Our bodies are designed to exploit the warmth and light of the sun while awake and to use the dark of night as a time of restoration and energy conservation. These established patterns remain to this day, guiding the timing of when you feel sleepy and when you feel alert, as well as when your body performs certain functions.

The other process governing sleep, called homeostasis, encompasses an internal drive toward balance and equilibrium that makes your body feel tired after being awake all day and refreshed after being asleep all night.

ANIMALS AND SLEEP

Although spending one-third of your life asleep might sound like a lot, you actually sleep less than many animals. (Cat owners know this well.) Compared with other primates, humans spend more time awake, which could have been an evolutionary advantage for early people, giving them more time to find food, protect themselves from predators and develop social structures.

Meat-eating species (carnivores) tend to sleep longer than plant-eaters (herbivores), especially the large herbivores. These big plant-eaters can't easily hide when they sleep, so they need to be on constant watch for enemies. A giraffe sleeps less than 2 hours a day, while the lion that hunts it sleeps more than 13.

Horses, known for being skittish and constantly wary of being attacked, sleep less than four hours a day. Their bodies are adapted to doze while standing up: Tendons and ligaments in their legs essentially have a lock position that keeps them upright during light sleep. For deeper, more active sleep, they must lie down, so they spend only a few minutes in that stage.

Most mammals are polyphasic sleepers, meaning they wake and sleep repeatedly, sometimes around the clock, although some may favor day and others night. Sleep poses special prob-

In a daily dance, these two forces step to the forefront or recede to the background at carefully choreographed times to make you feel appropriately sleepy or fittingly alert. (You'll learn more about them later in this book.) During the part of this dance when you're asleep, a lot is going on.

Body restoration and hormone release
After the wear and tear of a long day, your body basically becomes a repair shop at night. Cellular division to regrow damaged tissue kicks

---

lems for certain types of creatures: Mammals that live in water risk drowning, while birds that stay aloft for long periods might fly into something or simply plummet from the sky. To solve these problems, some animals evolved to sleep with only half their brain on at a time.

During migration, some species of birds fly for many days straight. Bird evolution solved this problem by having only half their brain fall asleep, while the other half stays awake and vigilant. Some whales and dolphins, which must breathe at the surface, also never enter deep sleep with both halves of their brain at once. Because deep sleep can be so difficult to wake from, one hemisphere of their brain remains awake to prevent drowning.

Not all species experience the stage of sleep conducive to dreaming, but many do. If you have a dog, you've probably wondered about its dreams, which can often be accompanied by whimpering and the paddling of feet. In a process similar to that in humans, the brain of a dog switches off most muscle control while dreaming so that the dog can't act out its dreams. Some muscles are still workable, however, including those in the face, paws and tail — the parts of the dog that you see moving as it dreams.

into high gear, and healing processes peak. Stem cells, the raw materials that form different parts of your body, go to work, producing blood cells, growing hair, regrowing nerve cells and more.

At the same time, hormones — which act as internal messengers — surge through your body, triggering and implementing several important processes and functions. Growth hormone, well known for helping children achieve their full height, continues to be released during sleep throughout your life, though its levels start to decline beginning in your 30s and 40s. This hormone plays a key role in helping to maintain a healthy metabolism, control body fat and restore tissues. The nightly blast of growth hormone is so important that your body wastes little time delivering it into your bloodstream, with one of the most significant releases coming during the night's first round of deep sleep.

Sleep is also key to the production of two hormones that work in tandem to regulate your appetite by making you feel either hungry or full. The hormone leptin, which makes you feel full and suppresses appetite, increases during sleep, allowing you to go several hours without being disturbed by hunger. At the same time, ghrelin, a hormone that makes you feel hungry, is kept in check. But poor sleep can upset this balance, driving down levels of leptin (the "I feel full" hormone) and boosting levels of ghrelin (the "I'm hungry" hormone). The imbalance can leave you feeling unsatisfied after eating, potentially contributing to nagging hunger and putting you at increased risk of obesity.

Several other hormones are released during sleep as well, including melatonin, which is synced by the light of day and the dark of night; thyroid-stimulating hormone, which governs your body's metabolic rate; and cortisol, which helps you respond to stress. Adjustments to these chemical messengers are another important function of sleep.

Strengthening your disease defense

Sleep is crucial to a healthy immune system. It boosts your ability to fight off disease and infection. And when you're sick, it allows you to heal and recover.

A significant body of research has demonstrated that a good night's sleep helps fend off common maladies, such as a cold. In one well-known study, 153 healthy people had the virus that causes the common cold sprayed up their noses. Those who got less than seven hours of sleep over the following days were almost three times more likely to develop a cold than those who slept at least eight hours. Bolstered by a good night's sleep, the latter group's immune systems were better able to fend off the viral invasion and prevent a cold.

Sleep also can help you heal when you do get sick. When you're ill, you may experience an overwhelming urge to sleep. This is your body prodding you to let it devote more energy to fighting an infection. Because your immune system response is most active during deep sleep, when you're sick it's common to spend more time than normal in deep sleep and less time in other phases. This relationship between adequate sleep and a healthy immune system is seen in animals as well.

Sleep helps vaccines work better, too. After you receive a vaccine — say, for COVID-19 or the flu — your body requires sleep to respond fully and build a robust immune defense. If you don't get enough sleep, your body produces fewer antibodies, the protective proteins that fight specific invaders. Producing fewer antibodies renders the vaccine less effective. Studies have shown that sleep deprivation before or after getting a vaccine can reduce by half the number of disease-fighting antibodies your body produces. So, when you receive a vaccine, prioritize getting a good night's sleep in the days before and after the appointment.

Emptying the trash

The cells in your brain work hard as they think, remember, sense the outside world and oversee your body's physical operations. Doing all that work consumes huge amounts of energy and creates a lot of waste. As that debris accumulates, it can cause a host of short- and long-term problems. During sleep, your brain seizes the opportunity to clear itself of debris by activating an internal power-washing system.

It wasn't until 2012 that scientists discovered this neurological plumbing operation, which they dubbed the glymphatic system. They found that when you're in the deepest stages of sleep, space is created between tiny blood vessels and certain brain cells, creating a network of channels through which fluid can flow to bathe each cell. This fluid carries blood sugar (glucose) and other nutrients to help feed the brain's enormous energy demands. Waste products produced by the brain are carried away in the same fluid current.

One such waste product is beta-amyloid, a sticky protein that can accumulate and form plaques in the brain. The protein is associated with degenerative conditions including Alzheimer's disease and other dementias. Research in rodents and humans indicates that beta-amyloid residue increases with sleep deprivation. Also, as you get older, this waste-clearing process becomes less efficient for several reasons, including a decline in fluid production and reduced pressure and pumping action.

The discovery of the glymphatic system has led scientists to begin searching for medications to regulate it and perhaps slow or reverse degenerative neurological diseases, including Alzheimer's disease and other dementias. In the meantime, scientists have begun to identify lifestyle variables that could affect the glymphatic system's ability to clear the brain of daily waste. Research suggests that the system may benefit from omega-3 fatty acids, found in fish oil and in some plant sources. Exercise increases the flow of the glymphatic system, and heavy alcohol use reduces its performance.

Making memories

It's easy to forget just how enormously complex the brain's memory system is. You must remember some things, but not everything, or your mind will be overrun with trivial details. Some things truly are best quickly forgotten, such as the color of every car you passed on the road. But other facts and situations are far from inconsequential and must be retained for future recall if you're to survive and thrive. This task of remembering some things and forgetting others is so complicated that your brain does much of it after you've closed your eyes and dozed off, providing the peace and quiet needed to sort it all out.

Making memories is a two-step process. First, facts and situations get written into your brain in a place reserved for short-term storage. Then, during sleep, they get rewritten in a different part of the brain for safekeeping. Importantly, they're put in the right context so that you can find them even many years later. This process is called memory consolidation.

As you experience the world, networks of cells in a part of the brain called the hippocampus go through physical changes that encode the information. During sleep, some of these connections are

GLYMPHATIC SYSTEM

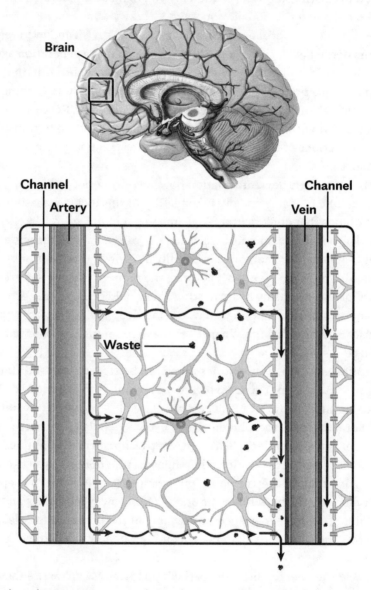

The glymphatic system uses channels surrounding arteries and veins to move fluid in and out of the brain while you sleep. Incoming fluid carries nutrients to feed brain cells. Outgoing fluid contains waste products, including beta-amyloid.

communicated to another part of the brain (neocortex), where they're added to existing knowledge, allowing you to make connections between old memories and new ones.

As part of this process, the brain appears to revisit and even replay events of the day during sleep. Studies done on rats a generation ago were among the first to show this. In those studies, neurons in the hippocampus fired in a certain order when the animal was running on a track, then fired in the same order as the rat slept. Researchers concluded that the rat's brain was replaying the sequence to transfer its recollections of the track from its short-term memory into its long-term one.

Because little new information flows in during sleep, it's the perfect time for filing and organizing. Part of this includes tossing away things that don't matter. With imaging technology, researchers can view how trivial memories are literally pruned away during sleep. Your brain encodes memories physically by growing connections (synapses) between neurons. Each day, the number of synapses grows enormously, increasing by up to 10%. This would be like a tree growing 10% more branches in a single day. During sleep, the brain does some landscaping, pruning the synapses to make room for new ones to form the next day.

Different types of memories appear to be stored away at different points during sleep. Those involving motor skills are enhanced during rapid eye movement (REM) sleep, the phase of sleep when the most vivid dreams take place. Memories of events, people and places are stronger after deep sleep. With age, deep sleep decreases, as does the ability to store memories. This suggests that doing all you can to get a good night's sleep remains important throughout life to keep your memory sharp. While your brain is filing away memories and learning from the experiences and events of the previous day, sleep also sets the stage for you to take in and retain new facts from the next one.

When you get too little sleep, the hippocampus can't write those short-term memories as easily and pass them along for long-term storage. Because of this, sleep deprivation can reduce learning the next day by up to 40%. Without adequate rest, your brain is simply unable to retain information as well as when it's fully charged.

Tempering emotions

At some point in your life you've likely gone to bed upset, only to wake the next morning and find you aren't nearly as worked up as you were the night before. It's not just the passage of time that tempered those emotions; this is also one of the beneficial functions of sleep.

One of the brain's remarkable survival strategies is to separate the emotional content of a situation from the factual content, then emphasize the factual aspect in memory, so that when you recall an emotionally charged event, the emotional punch has been watered down. Your brain appears to be set up for this, as some of the chemical messengers that accompany strong emotions are conspicuously absent during parts of sleep. Scientists have theorized that this nightly tempering of emotions allows you to avoid living in a constant state of anxiety, perpetually reliving traumatic memories.

Sleep also reinforces the brain's ability to be emotionally resilient. When you don't get enough sleep, you can become moody, irritable and overly emotional. Your thinking and reactions are more likely to be negative, with positive thoughts muted. Research has shown that the two parts of the brain involved in regulating your emotions, the amygdala and the prefrontal cortex, don't communicate well with each other if you haven't gotten adequate sleep the night before. This can prevent you from controlling your mood, as you might otherwise with the proper amount of sleep.

Basically, sleep provides emotional support in two important ways: helping you put what happened yesterday into the proper perspective, and preparing you to have a healthy response to tomorrow's events.

Conserving energy

During sleep, your body is conserving valuable resources. Just as many people turn down the thermostat in their home at night, your body dials down its temperature during sleep to save energy. Body temperature begins to fall in the evening hours, reaching a low during sleep a degree or two below its daytime peak. Your brain's temperature may fluctuate slightly during different stages of sleep.

In addition, your metabolism slows while you're sleeping, and your digestive system eases up. With all these actions your body is able to conserve up to one-third of its total energy needs.

BRAIN AREAS INVOLVED IN SLEEP

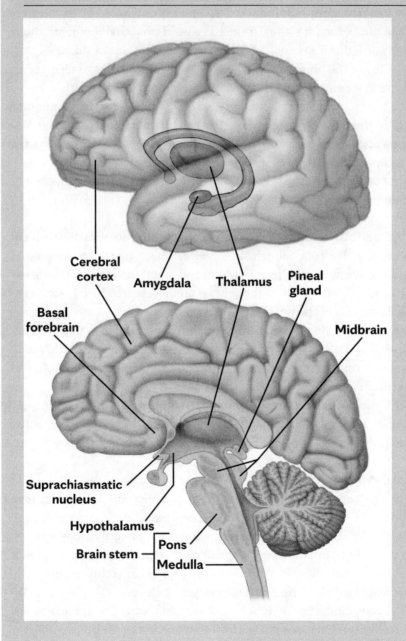

- **Suprachiasmatic nucleus.** This is where the master clock resides for your daily sleep-wake cycles. Connected to your optic nerves, it receives signals from the eyes about light and dark, an essential step in establishing healthy circadian rhythms and controlling sleep.
- **Hypothalamus.** Located deep in your brain, it controls sleep in several ways. Neurons in the hypothalamus produce gamma-aminobutyric acid (GABA), a chemical that helps summon sleep by slowing the nervous system. The hypothalamus also contains neurons that respond to hypocretin (orexin), a hormone for making you feel awake during the day.
- **Brain stem.** The brain stem connects your spinal cord to the rest of the brain. The brain stem is responsible for sending instructions for many of your body's most basic functions. It also takes information from the hypothalamus and sends out various sleep-related commands.
- **Pons and medulla.** Parts of the brain stem, they send the signal for your body to relax its muscles during certain sleep stages to prevent you from acting out your dreams.
- **Amygdala.** This brain region is believed to be responsible for the emotional content of your dreams.
- **Cerebral cortex.** It provides sensory content for your dreams.
- **Thalamus.** The thalamus largely shuts down during some stages of sleep, allowing you to block out the outside world, and gets busy again when you dream. It's also one of several locations in the brain that produce the neurotransmitter GABA to help sedate you during sleep.
- **Pineal gland.** Sitting just atop the brain stem, it receives signals from the suprachiasmatic nucleus to produce melatonin, a hormone that helps prepare your body for sleep.
- **Basal forebrain and midbrain.** These brain areas send signals to bring on sleep or to rouse you.

BRAIN WAVES AND SLEEP

Within the mass of cells that form the brain are some 100 billion nerve cells (neurons) that are in constant communication with one another. Brain neurons operate at lightning speed, allowing the brain to fire off messages from cell to cell instantaneously. It does this in two primary ways: with chemical messengers called neurotransmitters and with subtle electrical signals measuring just a few millionths of a volt.

A device called an electroencephalograph (EEG) can detect these electrical signals, which occur in wave patterns. Just like waves in the ocean, brain waves come in regular intervals and may be big or small.

The speed of your brain waves is measured by their frequency — how many occur each second — and that is expressed in hertz (Hz). A brain wave that peaks 20 times each second would have a frequency of 20 Hz.

Since the 1950s, sleep has been defined by researchers largely in terms of brain activity revealed on EEG, which shows that sleep is composed of several stages, each associated with distinct electrical patterns. EEG dashed the idea that sleep is one unified state of unconsciousness, instead revealing a wildly dynamic and multifaceted brain state.

As you might expect, your brain produces its fastest brain waves when you're awake. When you're taking in a lot of sensory information (sights, smells, sounds, touches, tastes) or when you're working to remember hard-to-recall things, your brain wave frequency reaches its peak.

As you become relaxed and drowsy, generally at the end of the day, electrical activity in your brain begins to slow. As you fall into the lighter stages of sleep, your brain waves slow again. However, you still experience bursts of higher-frequency waves that last just a second or two. In deep sleep, your brain produces its slowest waves. But during periods when you dream, brain waves speed up again, similar to when you're awake.

Early researchers determined that the brain typically produces waves in only a few different frequency ranges, which were assigned letters of the Greek alphabet as a kind of shorthand. These are the five types of brain waves:

- **Delta (δ), 0–4 Hz.** These waves, up to 4 per second, are the slowest your brain produces. Deep sleep is filled with brain waves predominantly in the middle of this range, usually from 0.5 to 2 Hz.
- **Theta (θ), 4–8 Hz.** Your brain produces these slow waves when it's relaxed and focused inward, including when you are in the two lightest stages of sleep.
- **Alpha (α), 8–13 Hz.** Alpha waves signify that your brain is relaxed and in a somewhat passive state. You could doze off at this point, especially if you're fatigued.
- **Beta (β), 13–30 Hz.** These faster brain waves are produced during much of your waking day and are also present when you dream.
- **Gamma (γ), 30 Hz or greater.** These are the fastest waves, produced when the brain needs to function at an accelerated pace to process large amounts of information.

In addition to these consistent waves, your brain produces quick bursts of electrical activity during sleep, called K-complexes and spindles. Spindles take their name from their resemblance on EEG readouts to spindles wrapped with thread, used in fabric weaving.

SLEEP STAGES: THE NIGHTLY PROGRESSION OF SLEEP

As mentioned earlier, sleep consists of several distinct stages. Similar to verses and choruses in a song, sleep stages usually follow a certain order and repeat (cycle) several times in that same sequence — or close to it. It's not uncommon for sleep cycles to vary somewhat, a bit of improvisation your body may perform with slight differences each night.

There are four distinct stages of sleep. One stage is rapid eye movement (REM) sleep. During this stage, your eyes dart about behind your closed eyelids. This is the time when you're most likely to dream, and you may dream vividly.

The other three stages are grouped together as non-rapid eye movement (non-REM) sleep. Non-REM stages are also referred to as N1, N2 and N3, with each successive number signifying a deeper state of sleep.

During healthy sleep, you progressively cycle through these distinct stages, typically four or five times every night. Each cycle averages 90 to 110 minutes, though the cycles can be much longer.

As these stages repeat through the night, REM sleep constitutes about 25% of total sleep time and the others split the remaining 75%. Early in your sleep, you pack in more of the important deep sleep stage, which then decreases through the night. Late in your sleep, REM sleep becomes dominant.

The amount of time spent in each stage can depend on different factors. REM sleep is largely governed by your circadian rhythms, so it tends to follow an internal clock and happen at the same time no matter what. The other stages are strongly influenced by the body's drive to maintain a balance of sleep and wakefulness (homeostasis). So, for example, if you go to bed after too little sleep the previous night, your body may respond by having more deep sleep.

Throughout the night, electrical signaling systems in your brain set the tempo and conduct the show. Chemical substances known as neurotransmitters that your brain uses for its internal communication rise and fall to accompany the different stages of sleep. Each sleep stage is important and plays a vital role in your well-being, and none is necessarily better than any of the others. All sleep is good for you!

Non-REM stage 1 (N1)

This first stage of sleep is so light that it might not seem like sleep at all. It's a transitional state between two worlds, sleep and wakefulness, and you may not feel you're entirely in one or the other.

This lightest stage of sleep known as N1 lasts only a short time, usually just 1 to 7 minutes, or about 5% of the sleep cycle. It doesn't take much to rouse you back to full wakefulness when you're in this sleep stage.

Physically, your breathing is regular and your body is generally still, though it maintains muscle tone and might twitch now and then. As you settle into sleep, low-frequency alpha brain waves, the sign of a relaxed state, give way to even slower theta waves.

If nothing disturbs you, you'll typically pass swiftly through this stage to N2 sleep.

Non-REM stage 2 (N2)
As you progress toward deeper sleep, your heart rate and body temperature drop and your muscles relax. It's more difficult to wake you during this phase than it was during the lightest stage of sleep.

Early in the night, the N2 stage generally lasts 10 to 25 minutes, but it grows longer with each passing cycle. By the time you wake, you'll likely have spent up to half the night in this stage, more than in any other. As you age, you spend even more of your sleep in N2 and less in deep sleep.

SPLITTING THE NIGHT: 'FIRST' AND 'SECOND' SLEEP

In the long span of human history before artificial light, the sun largely determined when people went to bed at night and rose in the morning. After all, it's difficult to get much work done in the dark. During certain times of the year in more northerly locations, darkness lasts significantly longer than most people sleep. Some people responded to this by going to bed when it got dark, waking in the night for a period of hours and then going back to sleep again before sunrise.

Ancient texts from various cultures contain references to "first sleep" and "second sleep," with a period of activity in between. These writings describe people socializing with neighbors, doing chores such as chopping wood, or eating another meal.

Scholars disagree on how widespread the practice was. Some believe it was most common only where winter nights were long, such as northern Europe.

The notion that two-part (biphasic) sleep may be natural and even good for you pops up occasionally in the popular press or on social media. Evidence for its benefits is thin, however, and attempting to wake in the night to get things done risks upsetting your body's internal clock (circadian rhythms) and can leave you sleep-deprived.

In this phase, your brain waves have slowed, but there are occasional eruptions of electrical activity that last but a second or two. These bursts — called spindles and K-complexes — remain something of a puzzle to scientists but are believed to play a role in storage of long-term memories.

It's in this stage, along with REM sleep, that experiences of the day are consolidated into your existing network of knowledge so that you can recall them later. This consolidation is a key step in the formation of long-term memories.

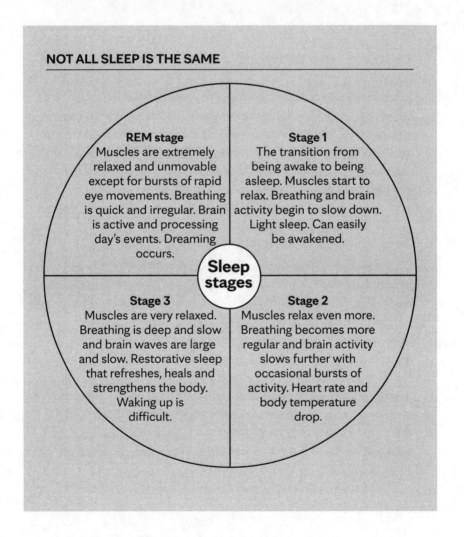

NOT ALL SLEEP IS THE SAME

Sleep stages

REM stage
Muscles are extremely relaxed and unmovable except for bursts of rapid eye movements. Breathing is quick and irregular. Brain is active and processing day's events. Dreaming occurs.

Stage 1
The transition from being awake to being asleep. Muscles start to relax. Breathing and brain activity begin to slow down. Light sleep. Can easily be awakened.

Stage 3
Muscles are very relaxed. Breathing is deep and slow and brain waves are large and slow. Restorative sleep that refreshes, heals and strengthens the body. Waking up is difficult.

Stage 2
Muscles relax even more. Breathing becomes more regular and brain activity slows further with occasional bursts of activity. Heart rate and body temperature drop.

While N2 isn't the most restorative stage of sleep, it does leave you feeling refreshed and alert.

Non-REM stage 3 (N3)

You enter your deepest sleep during N3, with the longest stretch — 20 to 40 minutes — coming in the first sleep cycle of the night. This could be an indication of its high value: Your body doesn't want to gamble on you missing out on this restorative phase of sleep in the event you're awakened during the night and your overall time asleep is cut short. On average, 20% to 25% of sleep is spent in this stage. As you age, the time spent in deep sleep diminishes, replaced by lighter N2 sleep.

You produce your slowest brain waves during N3 sleep, which is sometimes called slow-wave sleep. A brain wave may come only once per second, or even less frequently, compared with more than 30 per second when you're awake and deep in thought.

Deep sleep is a time for restoration of your brain and body. Your immune system receives a boost, letting loose the cells that hunt infectious viruses and bacteria. The body's repair processes are at work, including the release of growth hormone, which surges during deep sleep, especially early in the night. Your brain's glymphatic system also conducts its vital cleanup during deep sleep. Cerebrospinal fluid floods into your brain, washing away harmful protein wastes that accumulated during the day and offering a fresh supply of nutrients.

As a sign of deep sleep's high value, your body will try to make up for missed deep sleep the following night in what's sometimes called slow-wave sleep rebound. It's difficult to be roused from this stage, and someone who does wake up during deep sleep might not think clearly for up to an hour, their brain clouded by sleep inertia. If you sleepwalk, it's most likely to happen during this stage.

Sleep studies indicate that people often pass into this deep stage of sleep from the lighter N2 stage, then pass back into N2 before progressing to REM sleep.

REM sleep

About a quarter of each night is spent in rapid eye movement sleep, which is when most dreams unfold. It gets its name from the observation that your eyes dart about behind the lids during this stage of sleep.

Except for your eyes and the muscles used to breathe, your movement has nearly ceased. The brain stem has cut back muscle tone, bringing a temporary paralysis (atonia) that prevents your body from acting out your dreams.

Most of the dreams that you remember likely occurred during REM sleep. You can dream during other stages of sleep, too, but REM sleep tends to produce the most vivid dreams.

REM sleep typically begins about 90 minutes after you fall asleep and lasts about 10 minutes in the first cycle. Its length increases with each successive cycle through the night, with your final REM cycle lasting up to an hour. This can often be your last sleep stage of the night. If you don't use an alarm clock and wake naturally after a full night's sleep, it's often from REM.

During REM sleep, your breathing rate increases and can be more erratic than in previous sleep stages. Heart rate and blood pressure rise, and the brain is so busy that its electrical activity can look similar to when you're awake. Because the brain in REM sleep can so closely resemble an awake brain, it's sometimes called paradoxical sleep.

In addition to generating dreams, your brain does a lot of work helping to maintain your emotional well-being during REM sleep. The amygdala, the brain's control center for fear and emotions, becomes highly active during REM. This is when emotional memories are stored away and processed, often rendering them less intense and easier to accept the next morning than before you went to bed.

REM sleep helps maintain the brain's prefrontal cortex, which plays a key role in impulse control and decision-making. This part of the brain doesn't fully develop until after adolescence, partly explaining poor decisions sometimes made by young people. Research shows that when REM sleep is denied in adults, they, too, tend to make poor decisions.

SLEEP AND DREAMS

Dreams hold mysteries for the dreamer and the scientist alike. Both have long searched for the purpose of the strange visions, fantastic ideas and odd stories that unfold in the night. Dreams can be as emotionally potent as they are absurd, seeming to hold truths even though they're clearly untethered from reality.

Ancient cultures sought to find meaning in dreams, believing they were a gateway to the divine. Evidence dating back thousands of years reveals people seeking to encourage and incubate dreams to gain access to the important messages they supposedly held.

Sigmund Freud, the founder of psychoanalysis, is perhaps best known for popularizing a scientific — or perhaps quasi-scientific — view that dreams offered a window into the subconscious mind and were therefore key to diagnosing and treating several mental disorders. His classic 1899 book, "The Interpretation of Dreams," cemented in the public's mind the idea that dreams held meaning that could be unraveled to explain our inner thoughts.

That view began to fade with the discovery of REM sleep in the 1950s, which ushered in a new era of physiological exploration of dreaming. Dream research has only become more sophisticated with advances in imaging technology and the increasing power of EEG

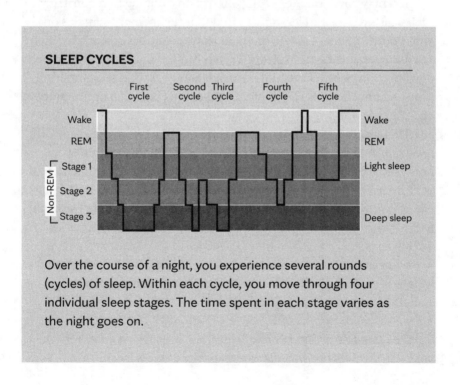

Over the course of a night, you experience several rounds (cycles) of sleep. Within each cycle, you move through four individual sleep stages. The time spent in each stage varies as the night goes on.

Understanding sleep   31

devices. In 2023, the National Institutes of Health Library cataloged hundreds of research articles on dreaming. However, despite the growing ability to peer inside the living, sleeping brain, dreams remain something of an enigma, their full meaning still elusive.

For decades it was widely believed that dreams occurred only in REM sleep. However, most people who are awakened from other sleep stages also report dreams, and people deprived of REM sleep still dream. It's now accepted that dreams can occur in any stage of sleep, though most tend to play out in REM sleep. Dreams that occur during REM sleep also tend to be more plot-driven and organized, even if they defy the rules of the real world. Dreams during other stages of sleep are typically vaguer, more like a thought than a little movie.

People typically dream about two hours each night, though they may be able to recall only a fragment or two of what they dreamed once they wake. Women are more likely than men to remember their dreams and nightmares, and for both sexes the ability to recall dreams diminishes with age.

You may have tried to recall your dreams, hoping to reconstruct their scattered narratives, only to find that the memory scurries off and is quickly gone. Certain brain neurotransmitters essential to memory diminish during REM sleep, so your brain is unable to recall much of what transpires. This could be an advantage, in that remembering those dreamy fictions too vividly could cause confusion between them and the real world.

There is, however, often some connection between the real world and your dreams. One theory of dreams is called the continuity hypothesis, which is based on the idea that dreams are a continuation of your daily life. You've likely noticed that significant events of the day can become incorporated into your dream life, and by some estimates, half of your dreams at night contain some element of the previous day's events.

Something that happened during the day that carried emotional weight is more likely to make the cut for your dream playlist than something that was less emotionally potent, even if that event was ultimately more significant.

One possible explanation for why your dreams include a rehash of your day involves the way that memories are made. During sleep, your brain is busy consolidating recollections of the day into your network of long-term memories. As you read earlier, your brain physically replays the events, with neurons firing during sleep in the same pattern in which they fired when you were experiencing the event. The fact that those events are also popping up in your dream life suggests that dreams are somehow related to that process. Some researchers, however, take a bit of a different view, speculating that dreams may simply be the result of all the work going on in your brain and don't necessarily have a specific function.

LUCID DREAMS: WHEN YOU'RE THE GUIDE

While dreaming, you might become aware that you're not in the real world and that what you're experiencing is just a dream. Lucid dreams are those in which your brain has access to both your waking memory and the content of the dream. Sometimes this allows you to steer the narrative of the dream. About 1 in 4 people say they have lucid dreams at least once per month and that these dreams are often pleasurable.

Lucid dreams can be therapeutic for people who experience nightmares, for example, allowing them to moderate the content to make it less frightening. This phenomenon has sent researchers to the sleep lab to explore possible techniques to induce lucid dreams and to teach people how to guide their content. Techniques investigated include medications, sound or light cues, and electrical stimulation to the brain.

One analysis of these methods concluded that there isn't enough evidence to show that many of the techniques work. However, the method considered most effective at prompting lucid dreams is a technique called mnemonic induction of lucid dreams (MILD). It involves training that encourages you to wake after a dream and convince yourself to become aware when you begin dreaming again.

Dreams also aren't only about processing the past. They help you anticipate the future. Studies have found that up to a quarter of dreams look ahead, not backward, in time. These forward-looking dreams, which tend to occur later in the night, may include fragments of past events and could be helping you prepare emotionally for the upcoming day.

WHAT'S ENOUGH SLEEP?

Sleep is a fascinating and complex phenomenon. Many of its mysteries remain; however, researchers are gradually learning more about the functions of sleep and its importance to our health and well-being.

One long-standing question is how much sleep is enough. This becomes an increasingly urgent public health question as the number of hours people invest in sleep each night is declining, not only in the United States but around the world as well. In the next chapter, we explore how scientists have answered that question to determine the amount of sleep you need to stay healthy and feeling your best.

2

How much sleep do you need?

If you're getting enough of it, sleep will consume nearly one-third of your life. That's more time than you will spend doing anything else. It can be tempting to look at all those precious hours as a place to cut back so that you can extend your day to fit in more work, chores, TV watching or socializing. After all, we all could use more time in our busy lives. In the long run, though, there's a steep price to pay for that.

Sleeping too little for even a single night can leave you fatigued and irritable. You don't perform tasks as well, you're more likely to make mistakes, and perhaps you just don't feel quite right. Fortunately, these effects can be reversed with a night or two of good sleep. It's easy to pay back a small sleep debt that you owe your body.

Sleeping too little for an extended period, however, especially over many years, isn't so easily remedied. Inadequate sleep leads to small but important disruptions of your body's most basic functions, starting a cascade of stress that harms your mental and physical well-being.

The damage is cumulative and is associated with several specific diseases and disorders.

COMING UP SHORT

More than 80% of the U.S. working population wakes to an alarm clock, bringing an abrupt stop to their sleep. So how do you know if you've gotten enough? Depending on any number of factors — from what time you go to bed to how often your sleep is disrupted during the night — you may be getting enough sleep. Or it could be that you're shortchanging your body a bit, night after night. You'll learn how to gauge if you're doing OK on the sleep spectrum or if you could use more sleep later in this book.

Ultimately, sleep needs are as individual as any other human trait and vary from person to person — some people need more than others. But you shouldn't mistake how much sleep you *get* for how much sleep you *need*. Chances are pretty good that you're getting less sleep than your body requires for optimal daily performance and long-term health. About 30% of U.S. adults say they receive less than the optimal amount of sleep.

While some people may believe that they can get by on only five or six hours a night, they're likely mistaken. Just as someone who's had a few drinks might not be the best judge of whether they're impaired, a sleep-deprived person might not have a clear understanding of the significant ways their health and performance are affected by too little sleep.

Only about 1% of the population truly needs to sleep just six hours or less to support their physical and mental well-being. Scientists have identified a genetic mutation that causes this, which is why this short-sleeping trait runs in some families.

For those of us who fall among the 99 out of 100 people who aren't natural short-sleepers, it's wise to look at the experts' recommendations regarding sleep and understand how and why those recommendations were developed.

Individualizing how much sleep you "need" can be a bit complicated. As you'll come to learn, sleep needs encompass getting enough total sleep, getting good-quality sleep and getting your sleep at the best time for your body. Maintaining a regular sleep schedule is vital because your body thrives on consistency. It's better able to restore itself when you heed its internal clock.

MEASUREMENTS OF A GOOD NIGHT'S SLEEP

What constitutes a good night's sleep? It seems like a simple enough question, but the answer isn't always easy or straightforward.

A good place to start is to ask yourself if you wake up feeling rested and remain alert and energetic throughout most of the day. After a poor night's sleep, you don't feel well rested when your alarm clock rouses you, and you may notice you're not performing as well as you could. Using that standard to define good versus poor sleep is a sound beginning.

But there are other factors that contribute to a restful night, including how long you were asleep, how often and when you woke during the night, and even how well your brain cycled through the many processes it requires to become fully restored.

To better understand healthy sleep — and where it sometimes goes wrong — sleep experts generally rely on a few characteristics that they can measure and evaluate independently.

Key measures include how much time you spend in bed, how long you take to fall asleep, how many minutes you're awake during the night and your total time asleep. Additionally, these characteristics can be used to evaluate the overall efficiency of your sleep. Sleep regularity — going to bed and waking at about the same time each day — is important, too.

Time in bed
Ask someone how much sleep they got the night before, and they might answer, "I went to bed at 10 and got up at 6." However, that didn't really answer the question of how long they slept. Rather, they relayed how much time they spent in bed.

To gain a better understanding of sleep, scientists and doctors look at time spent in bed and time asleep as two distinct measurements.

Time spent in bed starts when you're in bed and trying to fall asleep, not reading or talking with your partner.

Time to fall asleep
The number of minutes it takes you to fall asleep is one factor influencing sleep quality. How quickly you fall asleep can be strongly influenced by your bedtime routine, including time spent looking at your phone or computer, and your lifestyle choices, such as when you last drank coffee or alcohol. Falling asleep within 20 or 30 minutes of going to bed is generally considered good. In scientific papers, the time it takes to fall asleep is referred to as sleep onset latency.

ARE SLEEP TRACKERS ACCURATE?

Perhaps you're one of the millions of people who go to sleep each night wearing a watch-like device that professes to monitor how well you slept. But do these devices really do what they claim, and are they useful?

In general, the devices are sufficiently accurate to help you gain some insight into your sleep and bedtime habits. One device was even said to have "high overall accuracy." However, you shouldn't use such devices to try to diagnose a sleep disorder such as obstructive sleep apnea or insomnia.

This technology, known as actigraphy, uses sensors and algorithms to translate your body's movements into measurements of sleep. These measurements include how long it took you to fall asleep, how often you wake during the night, how quickly you fall back asleep and your total time sleeping.

Sleep trackers are most commonly worn on the wrist while you sleep, but some versions rest on or under your mattress or beside the bed.

Research indicates that high-end, expensive versions of this technology used by scientists and doctors are accurate. One

Time spent awake

Waking up occasionally during the night is common for many people. However, waking up regularly to use the bathroom or because of loud noises outside or your partner's snoring can disturb your sleep.

Waking episodes can increase in frequency as you get older, a time when urinary issues and other health problems tend to become more prevalent. Stress and anxiety also can make it difficult to sleep and fall back asleep.

Some people simply aren't aware of how often they wake each night. This tends to be particularly true among people with obstructive sleep apnea. Sometimes the cumulative effect of these awakenings —

---

study compared results from polysomnography, the gold standard for monitoring sleep, with clinical actigraphy and found that on average the sleep tracker overestimated sleep by less than a minute. That number increased, though, to a more significant 25 minutes for people with sleep apnea. And it underestimated sleep for individuals with narcolepsy by more than 24 minutes.

Most consumer sleep trackers haven't undergone published validation, so their results can vary. The American Academy of Sleep Medicine, a professional society that promotes healthy sleep and sets standards for diagnosis, therapy and sleep testing, stated that while consumer sleep technologies shouldn't be viewed as a replacement for seeing a doctor, the devices might be helpful for keeping people engaged as they work to improve their sleep. The academy called for further studies, more transparency from manufacturers regarding the algorithms used and evaluation by the U.S. Food and Drug Administration.

In general, while sleep trackers do pretty well at calculating how much you sleep each night, they can fall short in revealing more subtle but important symptoms.

from when you initially fall asleep to when you get out of bed in the morning — can result in a lot of time in which you're actually not sleeping. Scientists call that time wake after sleep onset.

Total sleep time
Measuring how long you sleep each night is crucial to understanding how well you sleep. But identifying exactly how much you sleep isn't always easy. Remember, total sleep time isn't the same as the number of hours you spend in bed; it's the amount of time that you're actually sleeping.

Most of us aren't very accurate at estimating total sleep time. Studies suggest that people with sleep disorders are likely to either overestimate or underestimate how much sleep they get. Individuals bothered by insomnia are more likely to underestimate their total sleep time, while those with breathing-related disorders, such as obstructive sleep apnea, are more likely to overestimate it.

To get a more accurate answer, total sleep time can be tracked to varying degrees with electronic devices, ranging from inexpensive consumer products you wear on your wrist to a test called polysomnography, which monitors your brain waves and your physical state in a lab or clinic.

Sleep efficiency
One useful way to understand how well you sleep is to relate the time you spend in bed to the time you're truly asleep. The smaller the difference, the better.

Sleep efficiency is typically looked at as a percentage. If you spent eight hours in bed and were asleep for seven hours, your sleep efficiency would be 87.5% ($7/8 = 0.875 \times 100 = 87.5\%$). A measurement of 85% or better is generally considered good sleep efficiency.

Sleep efficiency doesn't take into account arousal frequency. An arousal is a brief transition of the brain from sleep to a wake condition lasting less than 15 seconds. If the sleep-to-wake transition continues for 15 seconds or longer, it's called awakening.

You have more arousals during the night than you may realize, and they tend to increase with age. For example, in a 40-year-old, up to 15 arousals per hour is considered normal.

Short arousals may signal being in an uncomfortable sleep position, or they may have some survival value, providing brief periods to assess the possibility of a threat.

Sleep regularity
As the science of sleep evolves, it's become increasingly clear that an essential element of good sleep is its regularity — going to bed and waking up at a consistent time each day. By sticking to a set schedule as much as possible, you can help your body stay in tune with your circadian rhythms, the 24-hour cycles that include signals when to be sleepy and when to be alert.

To measure this consistency, researchers sometimes track deviations in bedtime and total length of sleep. In recent years researchers have developed a sleep regularity index. Studies suggest the index may be useful in helping to assess risk of poor health outcomes.

Helpful but not definitive
These key metrics, while very useful, can provide only so much information. For example, they can't measure the length of each stage of sleep that you cycle through repeatedly during the night. Sleep stages are affected by a variety of factors, including health conditions, such as obstructive sleep apnea, as well as by use of alcohol and other substances. Also, your metrics change as you age.

Sleep stages, characterized in part by brain wave patterns, can be accurately measured only with polysomnography. Your doctor might recommend this test to diagnose obstructive sleep apnea, periodic limb movement disorder or narcolepsy, or to evaluate long-lasting insomnia or other disorders.

WHAT RESEARCH HAS REVEALED

For insight into how much sleep humans really need, health experts rely on scientific findings amassed by generations of researchers and scientists. Much of what we know about the need for sleep comes from studies of thousands of people followed for many years, sometimes even decades.

Studying large populations of people over long periods allows researchers to spot statistical trends that otherwise might not be apparent. One such study is a subset of the landmark Framingham Heart Study, which in the 1940s began tracking the health outcomes of thousands of people in the Massachusetts city that gives the study its name. From this research, investigators have amassed data that reveals hidden clues about healthy versus unhealthy lifestyle choices.

A sleep spinoff of the study — the Framingham Sleep Heart Health Study — began in the 1990s and concluded in 2010, focusing solely on the impact of sleep. It tracked the sleep and cardiovascular health of more than 6,000 people, resulting in more than 130 published findings. Results showed, for example, that sleep apnea is associated with cardiovascular disease and that sleeping too little increases risk of high blood pressure (hypertension).

Many other ambitious and notable studies also have contributed to the understanding of how much sleep we need. The Jackson Heart Study was launched in 1997 as the largest examination of cardiovascular disease in Americans of African descent, involving more than 5,000 participants in Jackson, Mississippi. The data led to findings that participants who reported sleeping either a long time or a short time had an increased risk of cardiovascular disease.

Studies that similarly looked at large populations of people also have identified connections between too little or too much sleep and increased risk of diseases such as breast cancer, colorectal cancer, obesity and type 2 diabetes.

One recent study of adults between the ages of 20 and 39 indicated that those who slept less than seven hours a night had poor general health and lower scores on quality-of-life surveys.

None of these studies is an outlier. All of them echo and validate conclusions sleep scientists and statisticians have been making for decades. Their value comes from being rooted in the real-world health outcomes of people followed over long periods.

Research conducted in a laboratory or under other controlled conditions has also helped scientists to better understand the body's need for sleep and what happens when sleep is cut short. For example, researchers have been able to observe and measure changes in specific functions, such as how the body uses insulin differently when sleep is cut short, or how hunger-regulating hormones increase when a person is tired, making the body crave fatty, sweet and salty snacks.

Because these sleep restriction studies were done for short periods, scientists can't say for sure what long-term effects too little sleep has on a person's metabolism. But when lab results that show changes in appetite and insulin sensitivity are combined with real-world studies highlighting an increased risk of type 2 diabetes, a fairly convincing picture emerges of how getting too little sleep can affect your metabolism in profound and harmful ways.

Whether it's in a lab or taking place in the real world, research findings tell a compelling story about the need for sleep and the mounting cost to the body when it's shortchanged. The data clearly points to a strong relationship between sleep, your overall health, mental performance and your risk of several specific diseases and disorders.

Using these and other scientific outcomes, experts have come to some agreement on how much sleep most people need for good health.

SLEEP RECOMMENDATIONS AS YOU AGE

From infancy through your senior years, your sleep needs change. The galloping development of the human brain in infancy requires long and frequent stretches of sleep. In the middle of your life, your sleep needs even out. In later years, you need just as much sleep, though it can become more challenging to get.

Relying on an enormous body of available research, sleep experts have carefully crafted recommendations for how much sleep is needed during different stages of life.

The recommended hours for children, which are endorsed by the American Academy of Pediatrics, are intended to promote the healthy development of the body and brain, including improved attention, learning, memory and emotional control.

Sleep guidelines for adults, which were drafted by the American Academy of Sleep Medicine and the Sleep Research Society, are designed to promote optimal health throughout life.

These are the current sleep recommendations based on age:
- **Newborns.** In the first four months, a newborn's sleep patterns are changing rapidly and will vary widely, so experts don't make recommendations for this earliest stage of life.
- **Infants.** From 4 to 12 months, a baby requires 12 to 16 hours of sleep each day, including naps.
- **1- and 2-year-olds.** As development continues and many children learn to walk and talk, they require 11 to 14 hours of sleep each day, including naps.
- **3- to 5-year-olds.** A growing child needs 10 to 13 hours of sleep daily, including naps.
- **6- to 12-year-olds.** In these grade school years, a child requires 9 to 12 hours of sleep each day.
- **13- to 17-year-olds.** Teenagers require 8 to 10 hours of sleep each day. Experts note that teenagers who don't get enough sleep are at greater risk of self-harm and suicidal thoughts.
- **18- to 60-year-olds.** Throughout most of your life, you need 7 or more hours of sleep. Young adults, people trying to make up for lost sleep and those who are ill may need more than 9 hours.
- **60-year-olds and above.** As you age, your sleep needs stay about the same — 7 to 9 hours each night. However, you might find that you fall asleep and wake earlier. You also may require more time in bed to get the required hours of sleep.

CIRCADIAN RHYTHMS AND SLEEP NEEDS

For centuries, scientists have observed that living things, from plants to people, follow a schedule that appears to be in sync with the Earth's day. But it wasn't until 1959 that Franz Halberg, a Romanian scientist working at the University of Minnesota, coined the term *circadian* to describe this and jump-start our understanding of how time is at work across biology.

Circadian rhythms are the physical and mental patterns that your body cycles through daily. Because this clock affects so many of your body's systems, disturbing its rhythms — or trying to ignore or defy them — can have serious long-term consequences. Disturbances to

RECOMMENDED SLEEP BY AGE

Age group	Recommended sleep
Newborn 0-3 months	Sleep varies widely
Infant 4-12 months	12-16 hours
Toddler 1-2 years	11-14 hours
Preschool 3-5 years	10-13 hours
School age 6-12 years	9-12 hours
Teenager 13-17 years	8-10 hours
Adult 18-60 years	7-9 hours
Older adult 60 years+	7-9 hours

How much sleep do you need?

circadian rhythms have been linked to increased body mass and waist size along with other risk factors for cardiovascular disease, including elevated triglycerides and poorly balanced cholesterol levels.

Your body functions on internal clocks working at the molecular level to time its processes and functions. Humans also have a master

---

CAN YOU GET TOO MUCH SLEEP?

Getting too little sleep is clearly associated with negative health outcomes. Sleeping too much has also been associated with an increased risk of health problems, but experts aren't in agreement about what this means. Cause and effect can be murky here: Does too much sleep lead to poor health, or does someone in poor health sleep longer?

Research suggests that for adults, regularly sleeping more than nine hours is associated with poor health outcomes, ranging from depression to cardiovascular disease and even death.

However, when the American Academy of Sleep Medicine set recommendations for sleep, experts determined there was little evidence linking longer sleep and poor health. The academy found "only a few studies demonstrating an association of poorer general health or increased risk/presence of disease with 9 [or more] hours of sleep."

Ultimately, the experts couldn't reach consensus on how too much sleep could be harmful. For that reason, their recommendations for anyone over 18 years of age include only a minimum — seven hours — and not a maximum amount of sleep.

However, there may be cause for concern if you're sleeping more than nine hours each night, or if you notice that you need more sleep than you used to. Either of these can indicate a physical or mental condition that may require treatment. If you believe that you're sleeping an excessive amount, discuss it with a medical professional.

clock made of some 20,000 neurons located in a part of the brain called the hypothalamus. This internal clock guides the body through daily cycles of sleepiness and alertness. As the length of each day changes through the seasons, your circadian rhythms reset regularly according to exposure to light.

The body's internal clock also governs other key functions, including body temperature, hunger and digestion, and the release of hormones. One of these hormones is melatonin, which promotes sleep.

While we all share these circadian rhythms, personal clocks can vary. The inclination to feel sleepy or wakeful at a certain time of day

YOUR BODY'S INTERNAL CLOCK

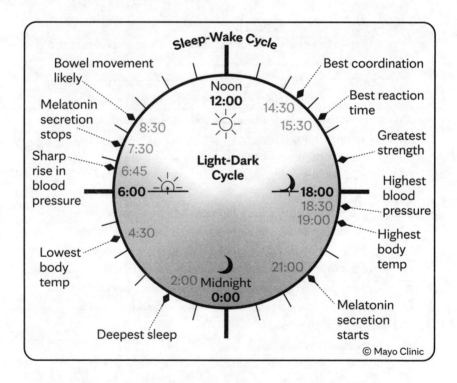

The sleep-wake cycle is regulated by light and darkness. The cycle influences several key bodily functions including body temperature, blood pressure and the release of hormones, such as melatonin.

How much sleep do you need?

ADJUSTING TO DAYLIGHT SAVING TIME

Once a year, a majority of Americans wake up an hour earlier than the day before. Each March we "spring forward" with the advent of daylight saving time, resetting our clocks from 2 a.m. to 3 a.m. This can be such a jolt to our circadian rhythms that it's now recognized as a public health issue.

Daylight saving was first adopted in the United States during World War I as a way to save energy. In 1966, Congress made it law.

Four decades later, researchers for the first time found that heart attacks increased in the first week after this springtime shift, especially among women. Since then, some studies have suggested an increase in heart attacks by as much as 29% following the time change. Other studies, however, have not produced similar results.

"Springing forward" has also been linked to sleep deprivation and fatigue, as well as headaches and reduced alertness. The change back to standard time in the fall, meanwhile, is associated with fewer health problems.

You can prepare your body for the time change by going to bed 15 or 20 minutes earlier each night as daylight saving time approaches. There are other things you can do to signal your body to begin shifting, such as eating dinner a bit earlier.

The American Academy of Sleep Medicine suggests the following steps to help handle this yearly springtime change, which occurs at 2 a.m. on a Sunday morning:

- On Saturday night, set your clock ahead one hour early in the evening and go to sleep when the clock indicates that it's your normal bedtime.
- On Sunday morning, go outside and get as much sunlight as you can. This will help reset your internal clock.
- On Sunday night, go to bed at your normal time, even if you're not sleepy and it feels too early.

is called a chronotype. Some people naturally function better in the morning, while others do in the evening.

As you pass through stages of life, your chronotype can change. Teens are likely to have a late night chronotype, while older adults are prone to have an early morning chronotype. Parents of newborns won't be surprised to learn that in the first three months of life, infants don't have a chronotype, sleeping and waking around the clock. Also, because men and women age in different ways, there are differences in how their body clocks change.

Morningness or eveningness: Which are you?
Some people naturally seem to be early birds, while others are night owls. In the 1970s, researchers set out to better understand these differences and invented words to describe them. Individuals who wake early and who generally think best before noon are assigned the trait of morningness. While they may think better in the morning, they're more likely to experience their peak physical performance in the afternoon.

Individuals who would rather stay up late and feel that they work their best in the afternoon or evening are recognized as possessing eveningness. They're most likely to experience their peak physical performance in the late afternoon or evening.

Researchers have developed a questionnaire to help sort people into one of the two groups. The questionnaire has been modified and translated into other languages over the years and is now available online. Questions on a typical test include:
- What time would you get up if you were free to plan your day?
- How hungry do you feel during the first half hour after you wake?
- If you have no commitments the next day, what time would you go to bed compared to your usual bedtime?

While the results generally place you in one camp or the other, they may be nuanced. You may receive a finding such as "moderate morning type."

Researchers have found the validity of the test to vary at least slightly around the globe, perhaps because of differences in circadian rhythm associated with the length of day at different latitudes.

Social jet lag: Is it affecting you?
Many people have experienced jet lag: After you fly from one time zone to another a continent or an ocean away, it takes your body's internal clock a few days or more to adjust. If it's time for breakfast where you have arrived but bedtime back home, you are more likely to feel sleepy than hungry.

What's called social jet lag has a similar effect on your body. However, it's caused not by airplane travel but by the scheduling demands of school, work or family. Even the decision to stay up late on Friday and Saturday nights to watch a movie or go out on the town can disrupt your circadian rhythms and lead to "social jet lag." The term was coined in 2006 to describe the lack of alignment between our daily schedules and our bodies' natural cycles of sleep and wakefulness.

Experts suggest that more than two-thirds of the people living in industrialized countries around the world suffer from social jet lag of at least an hour or two. That may not sound like much, but the health implications are potentially significant. Social jet lag is associated with increased risks for obesity, type 2 diabetes, cancer, heart disease and Alzheimer's disease. It can affect your thinking and your overall mental performance.

An early start to the school day for teenagers is one of the best-known examples of social jet lag. Many teens' internal clocks allow them to perform best later in the day, not when the school bell rings at 8:00 a.m., the average starting time at a U.S. high school. A school start time that's too early may be one of the primary contributors to the chronic sleep shortage among teens.

SLEEP NEEDS IN TEENS

If it seems like your teen is living in a different time zone, you aren't far off the mark. Teens are often driven by a body clock set differently than their parents'. This can cause conflict at home and be a drag on performance at school.

During adolescence, the body shifts toward an evening chronotype, so teens feel more awake at night and don't get sleepy until late. Because they need up to nine hours of sleep each night, their bodies are telling them to wake up later, a drive that collides head-on with the early start of school. One group of researchers summed it up by saying that teenagers waking at 7 a.m. for school is the equivalent of their 50-year-old teacher waking at 4:30 a.m.

Sleep is especially important during these formative years when the brain and body are rapidly maturing. One landmark study found that two-thirds of high school students were sleep-deprived, with girls more likely than boys to be getting too little rest.

Phones and computers — central to many teens' lives — are key culprits robbing teens of needed sleep. Social media and other online sites are masterfully designed to grab attention and hold it, delaying sleep for anyone who logs in.

A study of more than 5,000 adolescents found that those who spent more than an hour a day on social media got significantly less sleep. Researchers determined that social media shortens sleep in a dose-response manner, meaning that the more teens use it, the less sleep they get.

Additional research indicates that teens who can keep away from computer and phone screens and follow a healthy bedtime routine enjoy significantly better sleep. Other factors associated with less sleep included playing video games and the use of tobacco and caffeine. Interestingly, the factor that seems to have the greatest influence on better sleep for teens is a bedtime set by parents.

If you're parenting a teenager, be aware that research supports setting bedtimes and limiting evening screen time as effective tools to help teens get the sleep they need.

SLEEP NEEDS IN ADULTS

While your circadian rhythms may not change much during your adult life, that doesn't mean you're free from sleep hassles. Any number of life challenges — from work stresses to the demands of family life to the onset of menopause — can interfere with sleep.

From your 20s into your 60s, you generally need seven or more hours of sleep each night for your long-term health and best daily performance. Many adults don't get that much.

Men vs. women

Sleep needs for women and men are generally similar. Experts have determined there aren't enough meaningful differences between the two to create separate guidelines.

Women, however, typically take longer to fall asleep than men do and are more likely than men to wake up feeling tired. There are also some subtle differences in how women and men progress through the stages of sleep each night. Plus, hormonal changes during puberty, menstruation, pregnancy and menopause can bring new sleep challenges for women. These are discussed in the next chapter.

When it comes to sleep disorders, men and women also display some differences. Women are 40% more likely than men to have insomnia and twice as likely to have restless legs syndrome. Men are twice as likely to have obstructive sleep apnea.

SLEEP NEEDS IN OLDER ADULTS

Your sleep needs don't change as you age, but individuals age 65 and older often find it harder to fall asleep and are more easily disturbed during the night. Certain sleep disorders also become more common as you get older, including obstructive sleep apnea and restless legs syndrome. The result is that older adults often get less sleep than they need to feel well rested.

The structure of your sleep also changes with time, which might affect the way you feel during the day. As you age, you tend to get less restorative, slow-wave sleep and spend more time in the lighter sleep stages. Rapid eye movement (REM) sleep doesn't typically change in normal sleepers.

In addition, the older you get, the more likely you are to shift to a morning chronotype, waking up earlier. And because sleep can be harder to come by during this stage of your life, you might need to spend more time in bed to reach the hours of sleep you need to help you stay healthy and feel good.

3

When sleep is interrupted

Sometimes in your life, sleep might come easily, bringing an uninterrupted period of rest each night. Other times, though, sleep can be elusive. You might find it becomes more difficult to fall asleep. After you do, you may wake up, perhaps several times during the night. And worries that seem distant or manageable during the day loom large at 3 a.m. When you're feeling anxious, your body switches to high alert, and the possibility of additional sleep slips away.

As many as 70 million U.S. adults regularly don't get the sleep they need. A number of factors stand out as among the most likely to hinder a good night's sleep. Many reflect lifestyle choices, including busy schedules, work commitments, screen time and use of addictive substances such as caffeine, alcohol and nicotine. Other factors that influence sleep are beyond your control.

Understanding these factors and their potential consequences for your mental and physical well-being is an important step toward managing them.

CONTROLLABLE BARRIERS TO SLEEP

Many hurdles that stand in the way of a good night's sleep are self-induced. In today's hectic society, sleep often isn't a priority. In fact, lack of sleep is so common it's become the norm. We tend to view chronic sleep deprivation as a part of modern life. This isn't good or healthy.

Several aspects of our current lifestyles contribute to this sleep dilemma.

Putting off sleep
Many people simply don't want to go to bed at night. Some procrastinate before they lie down, while others put off ending the day by doing things in bed, such as looking at their phones. Researchers have given this phenomenon a name, bedtime procrastination, defined as "going to bed later than intended, without having external reasons for doing so." In other words, you're not sick, you're not working late; you just don't want to close your eyes and end your day.

Bedtime procrastination is often one of the contributing causes of inadequate sleep. Interestingly, procrastinators know they'll pay for their delaying tactics the next day, feeling tired and irritable. Still, they hold back on turning off the light. Some people are better than others at being able to shut off the TV or put down the phone, a skill known as self-regulation.

A few simple things can help you get to bed and get the sleep you need. Beating bedtime procrastination can involve better time management during the day, especially in the evening. You might delay going to bed because late nights are the only time you get to spend alone. If that's the case, plan some "me time" earlier in the evening.

You may be putting off going to bed because you fear you'll be unable to fall asleep. In some cases this might indicate undiagnosed insomnia. Speak with your doctor if anxiety about sleep frequently leads you to delay your bedtime.

Societal forces and work schedules
What time you go to bed and awaken each day isn't always a matter of individual choice. Norms of 21st-century society hold great sway over how much — and when — we sleep.

Early starts to school days are particularly ill-suited to teens, whose body clocks typically shift to a later time compared to when they were younger. Commutes and work hours can be out of alignment with individual sleep preferences. This is borne out by the fact that nearly everyone wakes to an alarm clock to get to work on time. Working long hours also impinges on sleep. In general, researchers have found that the more someone works, the less they sleep.

Working off-hours and evenings, usually required of shift workers, can take an especially heavy toll. Shift work can force someone to sleep at unusual times, disrupting their circadian rhythms and putting them further and further behind in sleep.

Shift work has been linked to increased risk of heart attack and type 2 diabetes. Because it's also associated with several cancers — including colorectal, breast and prostate cancers — the World Health Organization in 2010 determined that shift work is probably cancer-causing (carcinogenic).

In addition to increased risk of disease, people who work 12-hour shifts as well as frequent overtime have an increased chance of making mistakes and getting injured at work.

Then there's the seismic disturbance brought on by the COVID-19 pandemic, which upset the foundations of work, social and economic life. Sleep disturbances spiked during lockdowns. Not surprisingly, sleep problems were higher among healthcare workers, especially nurses. Children were also affected: They stayed up later, woke later and spent more time in front of computer screens, often into the night, which can make it harder to sleep. The rate of sleep disturbances almost doubled, affecting nearly half of all children.

Today, great swaths of the workforce continue to work at least part of the week from home. While the long-term impacts of this societal change will take years to become clear, it could prove to have a positive effect on sleep. Many people working from home use the time they spent commuting to sleep a little later.

A recent study found that people who split the workweek between home and the office slept longer and better when they worked from home, leaving them feeling less sleepy in the morning. However, they were also less physically active, which could impact sleep and have other negative health effects.

WORKPLACE STRATEGIES TO PROMOTE SLEEP HEALTH

Certain professions require around-the-clock staffing. From healthcare to transportation, service industries to manufacturing plants, employees must work evenings and overnight, times when their bodies are telling them they should be sleeping.

It's estimated that approximately 15% to 20% of the full-time workforce in the United States participates in some form of shift work.

Shift workers are at greater risk for sleep problems and the health issues that come with them. A number of catastrophic industrial and transportation accidents have been blamed in part on fatigue. Additionally, fatigued workers are less productive and more likely to miss work.

There are things that employers can do to help offset fatigue risks and promote sleep health among shift workers, including providing education programs about sleep.

Other positive steps include:
- Promoting short naps during work breaks.
- Establishing fatigue risk-management systems and including fatigue-related factors in incident reports.
- Allowing workers to have an anonymous system for reporting fatigue-related incidents and near misses.
- Establishing a system to help workers with sleep problems see a healthcare provider or an accredited sleep center.
- Providing lighting and other environmental factors that promote alertness.
- Not requiring evening and night shift workers to attend daytime meetings or functions.
- Incentivizing use of public transportation and educating workers on the dangers of drowsy driving.
- Encouraging telework or rotating shift schedules to facilitate more time sleeping.

Screens

Reading a novel at night might help make you feel sleepy, even if it's a thriller. Reading the same book on your tablet, however, could leave you feeling more alert and make it more difficult to fall asleep. It's not the plot giving you a jolt but the blue light aglow on the rectangular screen you're holding in your hands.

From smartphones to televisions, flat screens that have become ubiquitous in our lives emit light from the blue end of the spectrum. In

MELATONIN PRODUCTION

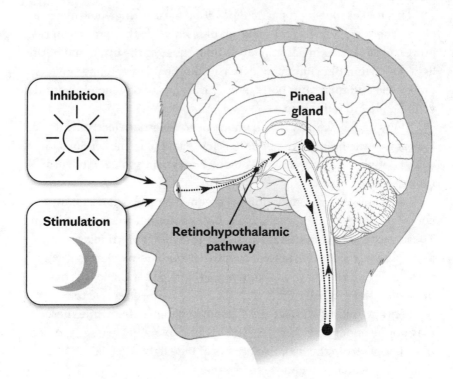

The hormone melatonin is mainly produced in the pineal gland. Its production is regulated by the retinohypothalamic pathway, which is influenced by darkness and light, including blue light from screens.

the past decade, scientists have become increasingly concerned about the potential for the light from these devices to interfere with sleep.

Your internal clock and the circadian rhythms that make you sleepy are set by the light and dark of day and night. When it's light out, processes are at work that keep you alert. When it grows dark, your body gets drowsy, urging you to sleep.

Your eyes send signals to your brain that tell your body when to start or stop producing melatonin, a hormone that helps you sleep. The brain tracts and eye cells responsible for sending these signals happen to be very sensitive to the part of the light spectrum that includes blue light, which is a significant component of the light emitted from electronic screens.

This makes blue light particularly good at resetting your internal clock. The wavelengths that make up blue light are three times more powerful at cutting melatonin levels than those at the other end of the light spectrum. Blue light can increase your heart rate, make you feel more alert and raise your body temperature, none of which is helpful if you're trying to fall asleep.

Many people who use a cell phone or some other electronic device look at it in the hour before bed. This has particular implications for young people, who may spend as many hours using social media as they spend asleep.

In response to our addiction to screens, some eyeglasses now come labeled as blue-blockers, claiming to filter out this harmful light. These glasses are sometimes touted for reducing eyestrain as well as helping you sleep. It's not yet clear whether blue-blockers actually work. Some studies haven't found any evidence that the lenses have an impact on sleep, while others suggest they may be effective for shift workers and people with jet lag. The bottom line is that while there may not be enough evidence to say that blue-blocking glasses protect most people from the negative effects of blue light, the glasses likely won't harm you if you choose to use them.

You also may find that some electronic devices now come with features that purport to cut back on blue light at night. Again, it remains unclear how much protection the features provide. A recent study of more than 160 college students found no difference in sleep among those who used devices with such features and those who didn't.

There are several possible reasons for this result. One is that while blue light can have a very powerful influence on the hypothalamus, it isn't the only signaling system at play, and blocking just blue light may not be sufficient. It also may be possible the filters aren't effective enough.

The surest way to prevent blue light from resetting your internal clock is to avoid using electronic devices in the hour before bed.

Caffeine

Having a cup of coffee is an important daily ritual for many people. Coffee lovers find satisfaction and comfort in the warmth of the mug in their hands, the aroma wafting up, and the slowly emerging sense that their physical and mental state is sharpening as they drink.

In the short term, caffeine in coffee can enhance some elements of mental performance. It can boost your attention and your brain's processing speed, and it can improve long- and short-term memory.

Caffeine also can enhance physical performance. More than a century ago, scientists published their first findings that caffeine increases the ability to do muscular work. Since then, coffee has been shown to improve aerobic endurance and movement velocity, which contributes to activities such as jumping, throwing or sprinting. It's one of the most common performance-enhancing substances used by athletes.

Not surprisingly, these perceived benefits can come with a cost. One short-term effect is anxiety and jittery feelings that can accompany caffeine use. More lasting, though, is the potential impact of caffeine on sleep. The sense of alertness that caffeine brings is real, and it can take many hours to fade and eventually vanish. Ultimately, this effect often bleeds into your sleeping hours.

Caffeine use has been growing, and the amount of stimulant in caffeinated drinks has been rising. Caffeine has had a resurgence in the marketplace, with so-called energy drinks and high-octane coffees. Along with these has come an increase in caffeine-related visits to emergency rooms.

Nine out of 10 U.S. adults have a caffeinated drink almost every day. By some estimates, the average person consumes 200 milligrams (mg) of caffeine daily. You might not even be aware of how much caffeine you're getting. Some examples: A 14-ounce Dunkin' brewed coffee contains 210 mg of caffeine, a Red Bull energy beverage has 80

HOW CAFFEINE WORKS

Caffeine's power comes from its ability to stealthily sneak inside the brain, where it impersonates chemicals that your body naturally produces there.

As your brain functions, it creates byproducts, including a chemical called adenosine. Your brain's signaling system has special receptors that latch on to adenosine. As adenosine accumulates on these receptors during the day, you grow sleepy.

Caffeine interrupts this normal process by elbowing the adenosine out of the way and latching on to the receptors. It usurps the position normally taken by the chemical that makes you feel tired.

Part of the reason caffeine can do this is that it's able to slip through the blood-brain barrier, a membrane of densely packed cells that keeps many harmful substances in your bloodstream out of the brain.

The amount of caffeine in your blood peaks about a half hour after you drink a cup of coffee, and then works for hours. The half-life of caffeine — meaning the amount of time it takes your body to reduce the amount of the stimulant by half — falls somewhere between three and seven hours.

An interesting question to consider is why as many as 60 plants, including those used to make coffee and tea, produce this weird chemical in the first place. Botanists believe the answer lies in the fact that caffeine is toxic to many insects and even some

mg, a tall latte at Starbucks has 75 mg, and a 12-ounce can of Diet Coke has 46 mg. Bang Shot, an energy drink, comes in at a whopping 300 mg of caffeine.

Researchers have long measured the impact of caffeine on sleep. One study that brought together all previous research reaffirmed

larger animals, so it serves as a line of defense for the plants. In other words, the active ingredient in that pick-me-up cup of coffee is in fact a mild natural pesticide.

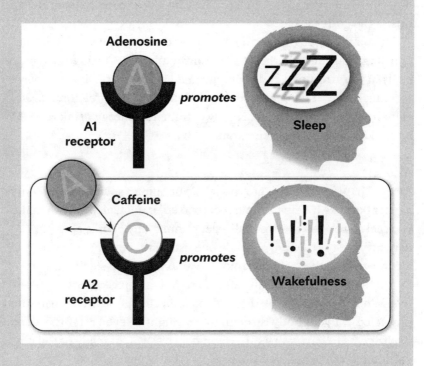

that caffeine consumption increases the time it takes to fall asleep, prompts nighttime awakenings and reduces total time asleep. The greater the amount of caffeine and the closer to bedtime it's consumed determine how many minutes of sleep can be lost. To prevent the caffeine in a typical cup of coffee from cutting into your sleep, you'd have to drink it more than 8½ hours before bedtime. A high-caffeine workout drink requires more than 13 hours to be cleared from the body before sleep.

Caffeine consumption can create a vicious cycle. You feel that you need caffeine to perform well and be alert. But at night you can't sleep from too much caffeine. Because you don't feel well rested the next day, you again turn to caffeine to function. Some researchers refer to this as the coffee cycle.

If you feel tired during the day or need coffee to get going in the morning, consider whether it's hurting your sleep. Cutting back, especially in the afternoon and evening, could leave you feeling and performing better. If you have trouble sleeping, avoid coffee for at least eight hours before bedtime. Highly caffeinated energy drinks should be avoided under any circumstances.

Alcohol

Alcohol has been woven into the fabric of human society for millennia, in part because it helps people feel relaxed. In fact, alcohol can make you feel so relaxed that you fall asleep, and many people come to depend on it for that purpose. By one estimate, 1 in 8 people use alcohol to help them sleep, ranking it among the top sleep aids.

In the end, though, using alcohol to fall asleep is counterproductive. While it can help you drift off, alcohol changes the chemistry and physiology of your body throughout the night — even after the alcohol itself seems to have worn off — and deprives you of many of the physical and mental benefits of sleep.

Alcohol is a sedative, slowing the workings of the central nervous system. It does this by altering the effects of several chemical messengers in the brain. Chief among these is the neurotransmitter responsible for inhibiting the firing of neurons, which has a sedating effect. Boosting the effects of this messenger — gamma-aminobutyric acid (GABA) — produces drowsiness.

Although you drift off, what follows isn't quality sleep. In the first half of the night after drinking, you fall asleep more quickly and slow-wave sleep replaces some of your rapid eye movement sleep. REM sleep comes later and lasts for a shorter time than it would without alcohol.

In the second half of the night, sleep becomes more disrupted. By this time, most of the alcohol has been metabolized by the liver, but the body is rebounding from its effects. Sleep in the second half of the night can become fitful as your body lingers in the lightest, least restorative phase of sleep.

Because it disrupts your sleep, alcohol can profoundly affect how well you feel and perform the next day. You may not be as alert and can't handle complex tasks as well. In some people this can create a cycle of sleepiness during the day, which is fought off with coffee, delaying sleep and inviting further alcohol use to bring on sleep at night.

Alcohol also increases the risk of obstructive sleep apnea by relaxing the muscles in your air passage. People who consume alcohol are 25% more likely to have sleep apnea than those who don't.

The closer to bedtime you consume alcohol, the more it affects your sleep. Some experts recommend a buffer of at least four hours between a last drink and bedtime. However, alcohol consumed many hours prior to bedtime, even during "happy hour" before dinner, can still affect your sleep. Avoid alcohol at night, and don't use it to help you sleep.

Nicotine

Nicotine use is on the rise, especially among younger individuals. Vapes (e-cigarettes) and aggressive marketing have created a surge in the market. Once you start using vapes, your body drives you to buy more. As the market for them has ballooned, vapes have become increasingly potent, loaded with more nicotine. From 2013 to 2018, the level of nicotine in vapes doubled.

Nicotine is a stimulant. Whether inhaled through e-cigarettes or from old-fashioned ones — or even consumed in chewing gum — nicotine revs up the body and pushes the brain in the opposite direction from sleep.

Using nicotine can affect the stages of sleep you pass through in the night, reducing restorative slow-wave sleep and rapid eye movement sleep. As with alcohol use, you're more likely to feel sleepy the next day.

People who use nicotine are more likely to say they have insomnia. That's because nicotine use cuts into the amount of sleep you get by making it more difficult to fall asleep and stay asleep. Smokers are almost 50% more likely to experience sleeping problems.

Nicotine is taking a heavy toll on the sleep of young people. Some studies suggest that 1 in 5 teens have vaped in the last month. While it will take years to understand the long-term health implications of this, one study found that teens who vape are nearly 30% more likely to have sleep problems.

If you try to quit nicotine, your sleep might become even more disturbed during withdrawal. You might sleep poorly and wake frequently. Some people also feel depressed. This can make it hard to quit. Hang in there! Many of these symptoms disappear within a few weeks of quitting.

Quitting nicotine is good for your sleep and your health. There are multiple options available to help you quit, and they can be tailored to reduce sleep disturbances as you go through nicotine withdrawal. Talk to a medical professional about which options would suit you best.

Worry

The relationship between stress and sleep — what's known as sleep reactivity — varies widely from person to person. A shared problem that might leave one person tossing and turning may have no effect on the partner sleeping soundly beside them. Researchers believe this trait is inherited, explaining some of the individual differences.

Certain life events are so stressful that they can be expected to interfere with sleep. A death, divorce, job loss or other traumatic development is likely to interrupt sleep for most everyone, even if just for a short time.

Your response to stress is mainly governed in the hypothalamus, an almond-size region of your brain where nerve cells (neurons) and hormones work together to send and receive signals related to some of your body's most important functions. Anxiety prompts a surge of stress hormones, including the hormones adrenaline and cortisol, making you alert and preparing you for danger.

One reason you might worry more at night: Your brain has less to do in the dark with the lights out, so it focuses on problems. More than 3 out of 4 people with insomnia indicate that stress is one of the things keeping them awake.

There are a variety of tools available to cope with stress. Sometimes expressing your concerns to another person helps. Other strategies include breaking big problems into smaller parts and making a list of ways to address them. Studies have found that people who spend five minutes before bed making a detailed and specific to-do list fall asleep more quickly than those who spend five minutes writing about their day.

Additional tools for reducing worry and managing stress include eliminating or cutting back on caffeine and using relaxation techniques, such as relaxed breathing, meditation and visualization.

Bed partners
Most adults don't sleep alone. Sleeping beside a partner is considered one of the most fundamental social interactions. Some biologists explain it in terms of evolution — in a world where predators lurk in the night, falling asleep can be dangerous, and being with someone else makes it a bit safer. The feeling of security that comes from lying beside a trusted partner can make it easier to relax and let sleep come on.

Sharing a bed can bring a host of other benefits. Studies have found that married couples who share a bed have more rapid eye movement (REM) sleep when sleeping together than separately, and they have more REM sleep than individuals who aren't married. REM sleep is an active stage of sleep where dreaming happens. It's thought to be good for mood regulation, memory and learning.

Some studies suggest that the benefits of sleeping with a partner versus sleeping alone might be greater for men than for women. One study found that men get more sleep when sharing a bed, while for women there's no difference.

Sharing a bed can bring disturbances during the night. Because people have different chronotypes — some are night owls, some are early birds — going to sleep at the same time can be difficult. According to some research, couples who go to bed at the same time are more likely to be disturbed during sleep than couples who choose bedtimes more suited to their individual needs.

Things grow even more complicated when one of the people in bed has a sleep disorder. Sleeping beside someone with a sleep problem can be considered a sleep problem in itself and can be harmful to your health and well-being. This type of sleep relationship has been associated with depressed moods, general unhappiness and an unhappy marriage.

A person with insomnia can disturb their partner, who in turn disturbs the person trying to sleep. This can create a cycle where both partners are disturbing each other. Obstructive sleep apnea, one of the most common sleep disorders, is often associated with snoring and frequent movements through the night. For the other person in the bed, this can be difficult to sleep through.

Individuals married to someone with obstructive sleep apnea have been found to be three times more likely than the general population to report difficulty falling asleep and staying asleep, two of the symptoms of insomnia. They're twice as likely to feel fatigued and sleepy during the day. More than half say their partner's snoring disturbs them almost every night.

For these reasons, treatment for obstructive sleep apnea can be life-changing for both you and your partner. Researchers from the Mayo Clinic Sleep Disorders Center studied 10 married couples where one partner had obstructive sleep apnea that caused disruptive snor-

NO INFANTS IN BED

You should never share a bed with an infant. Bed-sharing is associated with sudden infant death syndrome (SIDS), and small babies are vulnerable to being asphyxiated, entrapped or strangled in a bed with a parent.

The American Academy of Pediatrics recommends that for at least the first 6 to 12 months, an infant should sleep in a bassinet or crib in the same room as the parent, but not in the same bed. Some consider it safe to bring a child into bed at age 1, or as a toddler becomes able to free themselves from sheets or blankets.

ing. Treating the problem with continuous positive airway pressure (CPAP) reduced snoring, helping both the snorer and the partner get a better night's sleep. Using polysomnography, researchers found the snorer's bed partner gained an average of 62 additional minutes of sleep each night.

Seek medical help if you or your partner isn't getting the sleep you need. Because sleep problems are shared between the two of you, the potential stakes of doing nothing are twice as high.

Kids and pets

People don't just share their bed with a partner; many have a child or even a pet in bed, too. One survey found that nearly a third of adults in the United States sleep with a child, a dog or a cat at night. While there may be emotional or cultural reasons for this, such a sleeping arrangement often gets in the way of restful sleep.

Having older children sleep in bed with an adult is common around the world. Researchers in China, India, Japan, Korea and several African countries found that in more than 3 out of 4 households, children sleep in a parent's bed. Historically, group sleeping was a common practice, with many family members sharing beds. It's much rarer now in the United States, though more common among Black and Hispanic populations than non-Hispanic white populations.

The fact is, neither the parent nor the child gets as much sleep when sharing a bed. There may be cultural or psychological benefits, and many parents report their sleep is better with their child in bed, but high-tech monitoring says sleep can suffer.

One study found that children who slept in a parent's bed took longer to fall asleep, slept less, woke later and took longer naps. Even with naps, these children had less overall sleep each day than youngsters who slept alone.

Kids aren't the only ones to climb into our beds. Cats and dogs love to jump in, too. By some estimates, nearly half of the people who own a cat or a dog allow it to sleep with them. The trouble is, dogs and cats have unique sleep patterns that are very different from those of humans. Cats do most of their hard sleeping during the afternoon and become more awake at night. Dogs naturally wake several times during the night.

Studies show that when sleeping with a dog or a cat, you're likely to wake up more often and the efficiency of your sleep is decreased.

Many people find sharing a bed with their dog or cat delivers emotional rewards, but you might reconsider the practice if you have concerns about how long or well you're sleeping. If, on the other hand, your sleep isn't disturbed by your pet, there may be no need to evict it from your bed.

UNCONTROLLABLE BARRIERS TO SLEEP

Not all circumstances or situations that tend to rob us of our sleep are within our control. In fact, some of the major hindrances to healthy sleep involve factors we simply need to learn to live with and manage as best we can.

Age
Aging affects people differently. Some experience few, if any, disruptions in their sleep as they get older, while others struggle significantly.

With age, the body goes through several changes that can interfere with a good night's sleep. You might find yourself lying in bed with your eyes open before the sun rises, even as you desperately want to sleep another hour or two. Or you may continually hit the snooze button on the alarm clock, unready to face the demands of another day after a late or restless night.

There are many reasons sleep can become more elusive with age. Some of the more common ones include:
- **Health conditions.** The older you get, the greater your chances of experiencing a medical condition and taking medication. Both can affect sleep.
- **Circadian rhythm changes.** With age, the body's circadian rhythms often shift forward in time. Because of this, you may find yourself getting tired earlier in the evening and waking up earlier in the morning.
- **Sleep cycle changes.** How you cycle through the different stages of sleep typically changes with age. You may spend more time in lighter stages of sleep and less time in deeper stages. Because of

these changes, sleep often becomes more fragmented and less restful.
- **Hormone changes.** Production of hormones, such as melatonin and cortisol, changes with age, often disrupting sleep. The body secretes less melatonin, for example, which is normally produced in response to the onset of darkness and helps promote sleep by coordinating the body's circadian rhythms.
- **Slower recovery.** From jet lag to daylight saving time, the older you are, the more difficult it can be to adjust to changes that affect your sleep schedule, disrupting your sleep.

Gender

Women face distinct challenges to a good night's sleep, and many sleep disturbances are more common in women than in men. One reason may be that women often take on an inordinate burden of household demands, and some tend to put family needs before their own sleep.

Like men, women are affected by shift work that can interfere with their normal sleep patterns. But some research suggests that women are more likely to prioritize housework after working a night shift, while men are more likely to prioritize sleep.

Added to this — and perhaps one of the biggest reasons women struggle more to get a good night's sleep — are hormones. Hormonal changes can wreak havoc on sleep, and women experience several hormonal changes at different stages in life.

Menstruation

Cramps and hormone surges that accompany menstruation often aren't conducive to a good night's sleep. In the days before each period (luteal phase), the uterine lining thickens, preparing for a potential pregnancy. This is prompted by decreased levels of the hormone progesterone, which can alter your sleep architecture. During the luteal phase of your menstrual cycle, it's not uncommon to experience poor sleep.

Among women with premenstrual syndrome (PMS), the impact on sleep may be stronger. Some women report disturbing dreams, find sleep doesn't leave them feeling restored, and feel sleepy and fatigued during the day.

Some sleep disturbance during menstruation is normal. But if your sleep difficulties are severe and interfere with daytime functioning, talk to your doctor about options to help you sleep better.

Pregnancy
Sleep is critical before and during a pregnancy. It can affect your chances of becoming pregnant — too little sleep can disrupt the levels of reproductive hormones. Studies show that working off-hours, such as overnight shifts, also can lessen the odds of pregnancy.

During pregnancy, as your body undergoes dramatic changes, good sleep is important. But pregnancy can make sleep more elusive and less efficient. Researchers have called this the great paradox of sleep during pregnancy: You need sleep, but it's so very hard to get.

- **First trimester.** To sustain a pregnancy, the body produces hormones called chorionic gonadotropin and progesterone. These hormones can make you sleepy during the day and may prod you to head to bed early at night. During the first trimester of a pregnancy, you may find your body urging you to sleep longer, yet you still feel sleepy during the day. Your sleep might be poorer than it was before the pregnancy. This is partly because progesterone can both make you sleepy during the day and make your sleep fragmented at night.
- **Second trimester.** The second trimester of pregnancy may bring relief from some of pregnancy's uncomfortable symptoms, including sleep troubles. At this point in your pregnancy, you might not feel as sleepy throughout the day, and you may experience fewer nighttime disturbances, including needing to go to the bathroom or morning sickness (which can happen at any time of the day or night).
- **Third trimester.** In the final three months, sleep often becomes more difficult as your body accommodates the growing fetus. An increased need to urinate, abdominal discomfort, breast tenderness and heartburn all can interfere with a good night's sleep. More than 1 in 5 people in the last trimester of pregnancy get so little sleep that it qualifies as insomnia disorder. As you spend more time in its lighter stages and less time in REM sleep, sleep can become less efficient.

In general, some sleep disruption is common during pregnancy. If you believe your sleep is very poor, discuss it with your doctor.

Sleep disorders warrant special concern during pregnancy. Studies have found that people who experience obstructive sleep apnea during pregnancy are more likely to experience preterm birth, preeclampsia, cesarean section and a child with a low birth weight. And those getting less than six hours of sleep a night in the last month of pregnancy were found to be at increased risk for longer labor and cesarean section.

Insomnia late in pregnancy has also been linked to postpartum depression, the "baby blues" that can follow childbirth. Studies suggest that for some pregnant individuals with trouble sleeping, sleep aids may help prevent postpartum depression. But it's important to talk to a healthcare professional before trying any sleep aids, including nonprescription medications and supplements.

While naps can make it difficult for some people to fall asleep at night, during pregnancy they might offer some benefit to help offset the sleep disturbances that can come with pregnancy. Moderate napping hasn't been shown to impair nighttime sleep during pregnancy.

Menopause

Many women find they wake more frequently as they approach menopause, and the quality of their sleep deteriorates.

Hot flashes affect most women during menopause and can disrupt sleep. Estrogen levels fall, prompting the body's thermostat in the brain to become extremely sensitive. Even the smallest change in temperature causes it to pull out all the stops to cool you off. Your upper body suddenly feels warm, your blood vessels dilate, more blood flows to your skin and you begin to sweat. These hot flashes typically last just a few minutes but can continue for up to an hour.

Mood changes and depression that may accompany menopause can contribute to poorer sleep, too. Sleep-disordered breathing, which can include obstructive sleep apnea, becomes more common as well.

Sleeplessness during menopause can be complex, and in some cases it might be related to other changes in your health and life circumstances that can come with aging. That makes it especially important to discuss sleep problems with your doctor to find the best solution for you.

HEALTH EFFECTS OF POOR SLEEP

Poor sleep affects the entire body.

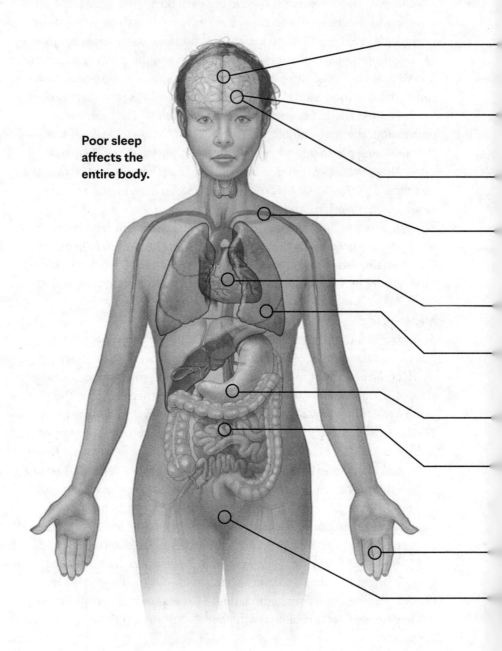

Mayo Clinic Guide to Better Sleep

Memory - Sleep is necessary for information retention. During sleep, brain cell connections are made to help with short- and long-term memory processing.

Mood - When we don't get enough sleep, we more easily become upset or irritated. Chronic sleep deprivation can contribute to anxiety and depression.

Thinking and cognition - Our ability to concentrate, solve problems and be creative decreases.

Blood pressure - Studies show that sleeping less than 5 hours a night increases blood pressure. Your heart beats around 100,000 times a day, so even small increases in blood pressure can have a big effect.

Heart and blood vessels - Lack of sleep can increase body-wide inflammation, which can damage the lining of your arteries and elevate blood pressure.

Immune system - When we're sleep deprived, we become more susceptible to viral illnesses, such as the common cold or the flu.

Metabolism - Sleep is necessary for healthy insulin and blood sugar levels, which reduce your risk of diabetes.

Weight - Lack of sleep affects brain cell transmitter signals that tell us when we're full.

Manual dexterity - Lack of sleep leads to drowsiness and decreased coordination, which can lead to falls and accidents.

Libido - Sleep deprivation decreases sex drive; in men, testosterone levels can drop.

CONSEQUENCES OF POOR SLEEP

As you'll learn in this book, sleep is central to good health. When your sleep is poor, the odds of developing other health problems increase, affecting virtually every system in your body. Inadequate sleep also impacts how well you perform mental tasks at work, at home and behind the wheel of a car. When you sleep poorly, it becomes harder to pay attention, your reaction time slows and accidents become more likely.

A sleep-deprived brain simply can't work as well as a rested one. Using advanced imaging technology, researchers can identify changes in blood flow in a sleep-deprived brain that mirror blood flow changes associated with declines in cognitive performance.

Insomnia and obstructive sleep apnea significantly increase your risk of obesity, type 2 diabetes, stroke, high blood pressure (hypertension) and heart disease, including heart attack.

Vast troves of accumulated data about sleep and health add up to one powerful statistic: People who sleep 7 to 8 hours a night live longer. Researchers describe it as a U-shaped curve, meaning that the further you get from 7 to 8 hours per night over your lifetime — getting either too little sleep or too much — the greater your risk of death from any cause. Some research suggests this may be especially true for women.

Experts also have come to understand that in addition to how long you sleep, the timing of sleep is important. Trying to sleep at times that aren't in sync with the body's internal clock can be unhealthy.

Performance and safety

Quality sleep prepares your brain to work well during the day. Sleep affects your ability to think, concentrate, learn and remember. And, of course, it affects your mood. Sleeplessness can leave you cranky and irritable.

Your body's ability to perform physical tasks depends on your sleep. Sleep affects reaction time, stamina, strength and speed.

In one study, basketball players who were encouraged to get more sleep saw their free-throw and 3-pointer accuracy rise by nearly 10%. They sprinted faster, became less fatigued and felt better mentally.

The data highlights the direct connection between sleep and elite sports performance. Other studies of athletes have shown they're less likely to injure themselves if they've gotten proper sleep.

Inadequate sleep, on the other hand, hurts your performance. As performance deteriorates, accidents become more likely. Driving becomes less safe. One estimate put the annual economic impact of accidents and errors caused by sleep deprivation at up to $56 billion. Much of that grim cost comes from the loss of earnings of people killed in crashes caused by sleepiness. Some estimates put the toll at 100,000 car accidents a year, resulting in 1,500 deaths, due to sleepiness.

Even a seemingly small change in reaction time can make a big difference in preventing an accident. In a controlled experiment, a group of French drivers in their late teens and early 20s were tested on their reaction time behind the wheel after sleeping either a full night or just two hours. With less sleep, the time they took to hit the brakes increased by less than a second — but at highway speeds, that translated into an additional 75 feet traveled by the sleep-deprived drivers.

The ability to stay in your lane while driving after a sleepless night is comparable to what it would be with a blood alcohol level of 0.05%. Most states consider driving with a blood alcohol level only slightly higher than that — 0.08% — illegal.

Potentially worse than slowed reaction times is the increased likelihood that you'll fall asleep. When your body is deprived of sleep, it responds by having brief lapses, or "microsleeps." These can last a very short time, even less than a second, as wakefulness and sleepiness wage a tug of war.

During such lapses, concentration breaks and you're prone to make mistakes. These lapses can become longer and result in dozing off. This can happen despite your best efforts to stay awake. If you're sleep-deprived and feel sleepy while driving, find a place to rest.

Obesity
Sleep can have an impact on your weight. A study that tracked a group of individuals for 16 years found that participants who slept five hours or less each night were 32% more likely to have gained more than 30

pounds over that period. As one researcher wrote: "The shorter the sleep duration, the higher the risk of obesity."

Experts aren't sure why there's such a strong connection between sleep and weight. It could be that people who don't get enough sleep lack the energy to exercise. Another possible explanation is that too little sleep can alter judgment, leading to unhealthy food choices.

When you're running low on sleep, you might feel the urge to eat more. In controlled studies, participants whose sleep was restricted consumed as many as 500 additional calories the next day. Research has also shown that individuals who sleep too little are likely to snack more often.

A possible explanation for this involves the hormones leptin and ghrelin, which are part of the body's hunger-signaling system. Leptin suppresses your appetite, while ghrelin boosts it. People who get too little sleep generally have decreased leptin and increased ghrelin, making them feel hungrier. In one study, participants who got just five hours of sleep produced 16% less hunger-suppressing leptin and 15% more hunger-boosting ghrelin.

Obesity is also associated with obstructive sleep apnea. This can create a cycle where being overweight contributes to sleep disruptions, and poor sleep causes greater weight gain. Losing weight through behavioral changes can improve obstructive sleep apnea and, in turn, bring health benefits due to a better night's sleep.

If you're overweight and don't sleep well, talk to your doctor about how the two might be related. Fixing one of these problems may help control the other.

Type 2 diabetes
More than 37 million Americans have diabetes, and the vast majority — 90% to 95% — have type 2. With this form of diabetes, the body becomes less responsive to the hormone insulin.

Insulin is critical to your metabolism, allowing the body's cells to access their primary power source, the sugar in your blood, known as glucose. When your body's sensitivity to insulin decreases, glucose goes unused, and it remains in your blood. Too much glucose circulating in your blood can damage nerves, blood vessels and organs.

The spike in type 2 diabetes among Americans is directly linked to diet and fitness, and the best way to fight the condition is to eat healthy foods and get plenty of exercise.

In more recent years, studies have also pointed to a connection between type 2 diabetes and too little sleep.

Individuals who don't get enough sleep have an increased risk of type 2 diabetes. In some cases, the risk was double for people getting less than five hours of sleep a night compared with individuals who got seven hours. One reason for this, as shown in lab studies, is that your cells become less sensitive to insulin when sleep is diminished. Just one week of insufficient sleep can leave cells 20% less sensitive to insulin.

Sleep disruption from obstructive sleep apnea is associated with insulin resistance, too, suggesting to some researchers that obstructive sleep apnea also may contribute to the onset of type 2 diabetes.

Good sleep is crucial to both preventing and managing type 2 diabetes. Too little sleep is associated with poorer blood sugar control and an increase in complications, such as kidney disease and vision-damaging retinopathy. An improvement in sleep, meanwhile, can improve blood sugar metabolism.

Cardiovascular health

Healthy sleep is important to your cardiovascular health. Heart attacks are more likely among individuals who don't get enough sleep. Some analyses of the data go further, asserting that lack of sleep causes heart attacks.

Sleeping too little can damage the structure of your blood vessels, including those that feed the heart. Insufficient sleep is associated with developing — or even dying from — coronary artery disease, a condition in which the heart doesn't get the blood and oxygen it needs. Coronary artery disease, which affects more than 18 million Americans, is the leading cause of death in the United States.

One study concluded that sleeping less than five hours a night was associated with a 25% increased risk of coronary artery disease. Several factors likely account for this, including the sensitivity of the heart to the body's circadian rhythms. When lack of sleep disrupts these rhythms, your heart pays the price. Inflammation may also play a role in how sleep affects your cardiovascular health. Levels of inflammation-causing proteins called cytokines rise when you get too little sleep.

Individuals who don't get enough sleep are more likely to have high blood pressure as well. The likelihood of developing high blood pressure increases by at least 60% with five hours or less of sleep a night. Women and Black populations appear to be at greatest risk for high blood pressure associated with lack of sleep.

Inadequate sleep also places you at increased risk of stroke. A recent study of people younger than age 50 found that risk of stroke increased 51% among people who had multiple insomnia symptoms, such as difficulty falling asleep and staying asleep, waking too early, or not feeling rested after sleep.

Following a regular sleep schedule that includes 7 to 8 hours of sleep is good for your cardiovascular health. One compelling study followed 2,000 people for five years, monitoring their health and the regularity of their sleep — whether they went to bed and woke up at the same time each day. Study participants who had irregular sleep schedules were twice as likely to have a cardiovascular event, including heart attack or stroke, when compared with those who followed a sleep routine.

The evidence is quite clear that getting a good night's sleep is one of the most important things you can do for your cardiovascular health, along with exercise and a healthy diet.

Dementia

Health experts are becoming increasingly interested in the possible connection between inadequate sleep and dementia. Several researchers have found that people who either don't get enough sleep or get too much are more likely to develop dementia.

It's also well known that people with Alzheimer's disease and other forms of dementia don't sleep well. This is likely caused by the changes in the brain that accompany dementia. Amyloid plaques associated with Alzheimer's disease affect the parts of the brain responsible for sleep and wakefulness.

It's difficult to untangle whether sleep problems occurring earlier in life were a cause of dementia that developed years later, or if the sleep troubles were an early indication of an already developing form of the disease.

Fairly recently, researchers discovered that one way the brain clears amyloid plaques is during deep sleep. Some researchers are exploring whether lack of sleep allows these harmful byproducts to accumulate.

A study that could help shine light on the question involves nearly 8,000 people in Britain who've been followed by researchers for at least 25 years. Findings from this research suggest that individuals who get less sleep during middle age are more likely to develop dementia later in life. And people in their 50s and 60s getting by on less than six hours of sleep a night may be 30% more likely to develop dementia.

Because this study reached so far back in time, some researchers suggest that lack of sleep is more likely a contributing cause of dementia than a symptom of the disease. And unlike some other studies, this one didn't find that sleeping longer than the recommended 7 to 8 hours was associated with increased dementia risk.

While more research is needed, what remains clear is that a healthy amount of sleep is good for your brain.

PAYING OFF YOUR SLEEP DEBT

Sleeping in is one of the things that can make weekends great. But if you think of sleeping in as a way to make up for your sleep deprivation, you might want to rethink your strategy. Research suggests that snoozing longer on your days off is a good thing to do if you didn't get enough sleep during the week — but the benefits only go so far.

Chronic sleep deprivation leads to many impairments — metabolically, cognitively and emotionally. Catching up on sleep over the weekend has been shown to compensate for some but not all of the harm done. You can't repay your sleep debt in full.

Sleeping in on weekends has some potential downsides, too. It can throw off your sleep schedule, making it more difficult to fall asleep during the week. If you do feel the need to sleep in, try to limit it to an hour or less to help maintain a consistent schedule of sleeping and waking. It usually takes a few nights of good sleep to make up for lost sleep. Researchers have shown it can take up to nine days for your body to return to normal after sleep deprivation.

The best strategy for your overall health and well-being is to get the recommended amount of sleep each night, preferably at the same time.

4

In search of quality sleep

Preparing for sleep doesn't begin when you put on your pajamas. Just as exercise and good nutrition should be woven into the patterns of daily life, your sleep will benefit from a consistent and thoughtful approach that touches on every hour of the day. You might sometimes hear these routines referred to as sleep hygiene.

ESTABLISHING A SLEEP ROUTINE

You probably have some good habits — and maybe some bad ones, too — when it comes to sleep. You may not even recognize them as sleep-related habits because some involve lifestyle choices early in the day. What and when you eat, the beverages you drink and how much physical activity you get all play a role in the quality of your sleep.

Of course, a healthy sleep routine also depends upon the hours immediately before bedtime. To optimize sleep, those hours should become a time to wind down, to slow your activity and begin signaling to your body and mind that sleep is coming soon.

The routines parents use to help children fall asleep hold lessons for adults, too. Putting children to bed is more successful when it involves calming activities, such as a bath and a book. Parents should put themselves through a similar decompressing routine a few hours later.

In many cases, improving your habits might require small adjustments, such as putting down your phone at 9 p.m. instead of 10 p.m. Others, including those that involve addictive substances such as alcohol or nicotine, might require your full dedication and consultation with your doctor.

The payoff for improving your sleep routine can be immediate. Feeling rested and alert the day after you take a deliberate approach to sleep can be an early indication that your body is getting more of the rest it needs. But this isn't only about quick fixes. Improving sleep can take time and a little trial and error, and it may require some modifications to your home and lifestyle.

Sleep requires time and consistency. It's impossible to squeeze in seven hours of sleep between midnight and 5 a.m. Your body also benefits most when your bedtime and wake time remain relatively constant from day to day. Both later bedtimes and variability in time spent sleeping each night are associated with worse health outcomes.

If there's one thing a century or more of sleep science has established, it's that sleep deserves to be a priority. We hear a lot about the importance of exercise for our long-term health, and everyone knows that diet and good health are inextricably linked. But sleep sometimes becomes an afterthought.

The topics covered in this chapter are useful for everyone. Even if you believe you sleep well, they can provide a tune-up. If you feel sleep-deprived, tired during the day, and know you aren't performing at your best, you could well find some answers here to help you. And for those of you diagnosed with a sleep disorder, the topics discussed here can help you form a foundation for good sleep as you work with your doctor on treatment.

As you'll see, developing good sleep habits doesn't need to be complicated. Consistently implementing many of the suggestions that

SMALL CHANGES = BIG RESULTS

Change can be scary, and it can be difficult to know where to begin. When it comes to implementing changes to enhance your sleep, understand that tiny steps can add up to big improvements. To make the process seem less daunting, take a small-steps approach.

First, develop a vision for how you want your sleep to be. Imagine when you'll prepare for sleep, when and what you'll eat and drink in the evening, when you'll wake up, and how you'll feel rested and ready for the day. Then take one small step toward that better vision, perhaps based on something you learn in this chapter. You don't necessarily have to do everything all at once. Stick with each small step for some time — say, two weeks if it's doing no harm.

If you see improvement, you're on your way. If not, make adjustments. Then look for the next opportunity to make a change for the better.

This small-step approach is sometimes referred to as *kaizen*, a proven method of positive change. Kaizen, which rose to prominence during the postwar industrialization of Japan, revolves around the idea that tiny measures can add up to big improvements.

The philosophy of kaizen — and of improving health — is to keep making small changes to your habits or behaviors that move you in the direction you want to go.

> Small actions are at the heart of kaizen. By taking steps so tiny that they seem trivial or even laughable, you'll sail calmly past obstacles that have defeated you before. Slowly — but painlessly! — you'll cultivate an appetite for continued success and lay down a permanent new route to change.
> —Robert Maurer, "One Small Step Can Change Your Life: The Kaizen Way"

follow could make a big improvement in your sleep as well as in your overall health and well-being over time.

Time
To begin planning for a good night's sleep, don't start by deciding what time you want to go to bed. Instead, think first about what time you want to wake up. By doing that, you can work out a schedule that accounts for the time investment needed for restorative sleep.

Consider how much time you need to accomplish all you do each morning. This may include caring for others, eating, getting to work

---

ZEITGEBERS: ACTIVITIES THAT AFFECT YOUR CIRCADIAN RHYTHMS

You learned earlier that light resets your circadian system, helping your body adapt to changes in the length of the day through the seasons, so it knows when to sleep. But light isn't the only thing that can reset your body's clocks. Your circadian rhythms are influenced by environmental and even social cues that ultimately play a role in when and how well you sleep by influencing brain functioning and metabolism.

In the 1970s, these factors were given the name "zeitgebers," derived from two German words: *Zeit,* which means "time," and *Geber,* which means "giver." Zeitgebers, then, are "time givers."

What and when you eat, for instance, is considered a zeitgeber. Your diet affects your hormone levels and your body temperature, which are keyed to your circadian rhythms. Exercise is another. It affects melatonin levels, one of the hormonal drivers of sleep. Other factors in your life, including family and work obligations, influence your body clock as well. These are referred to as social zeitgebers.

Being mindful of activities that influence circadian rhythms can help you to keep your body's clockwork in sync.

on time and other obligations. If you must be at work by, say, 8:30 a.m., and need two hours for yoga, showering, breakfast and commuting, then begin your sleep routine planning with a wake time of 6:30 a.m.

From there, work backward, building in the hours you need for sleep. Most people require seven or more hours of sleep each night throughout most of their lives. As you establish your sleep routine, you might want to block off eight hours for sleep. An extra hour in your plan gives you time to fall asleep and wake a time or two during the night, yet still get more than seven hours of sleep, as recommended.

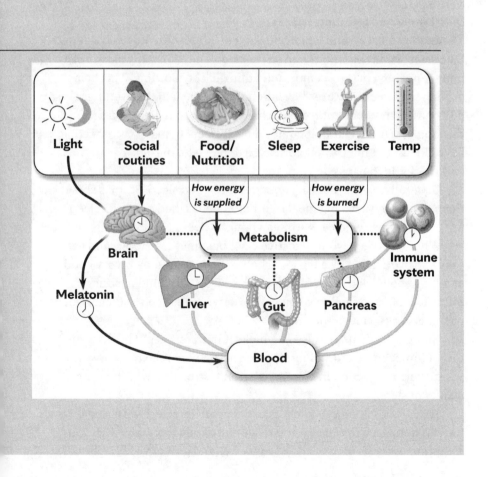

In this scenario, you would then plan to be in bed with the lights out, trying to sleep, at 10:30 p.m. You might have to adjust these wake and sleep times, setting them earlier or later through trial and error. Once you have arrived at what works for you, do your best each day to stick with the schedule.

Consistency and regularity are the foundations of good sleep. Your body lives by rhythms, and sleep will usually come more easily and be more beneficial when you follow your natural rhythms rather than try to ignore or defy them. Of course, there will be times when you stay up later, but try not to deviate from your routine bedtime by more than 30 minutes, or perhaps an hour, to best maintain healthy sleep.

Diet: Dinner and nighttime snacks
The food you eat — and when you eat it — affects the way you sleep. Like sleep, your appetite is tied to the body's circadian rhythms, with hunger peaking in the evening and falling in the morning. This helps explain why many cultures have their largest meal in the evening: The body has a large food intake, then has time to begin digestion prior to the long overnight fast that comes during sleep. In many cultures that have late dinner hours, people also go to bed late. In some cases, those cultures build in naps each day, too.

Generally, eating late isn't conducive to good sleep. Studies show that people who eat a big meal four hours before bedtime fall asleep faster than those who eat within an hour of sleep.

When you sleep, your digestive tract becomes less active and can easily be overloaded by a big meal before bed. Your body is very good at telling you if food is keeping you from sleep. From indigestion to reflux to a bloated feeling when you lie down, you receive signals when you've eaten too much too late.

Going to bed hungry also can make it hard to sleep. The discomfort of hunger and a rumbling stomach aren't very relaxing. However, a short-term reduction in calories or even fasting doesn't affect the quality of sleep.

Some foods are more likely than others to interfere with sleep. Researchers have found that the risk of insomnia increases with consumption of foods high in added sugar, refined grains and starches.

Fatty foods disturb sleep and can shorten it, and eating fatty foods at night is associated with weight gain.

As you develop your healthy sleep habits, consider whether eating or snacking in the evening might be disrupting your sleep or keeping you from falling asleep. Avoid meals or large snacks within several hours of bedtime. In some cases, that might mean you have a smaller dinner earlier, with a light, healthy snack closer to bedtime. A good nighttime snack could be a piece of fruit, for example.

Ultimately, the mealtime you choose will depend on influences as varied as your cultural background and your work schedule. Generally, an earlier dinner is better than a later one for promoting sleep, and it's healthier for other reasons, too. Individuals who have a later dinner tend to eat more and spend more time overall eating each day. One study found that for each hour later that a meal was consumed, carbohydrate intake increased 9 grams and sugar consumption increased 5 grams.

Alcohol and caffeine

If you consume either alcohol or caffeine, give careful consideration to how these substances could be affecting your sleep. Both have a profound impact on sleep, even when consumed hours before bedtime.

Caffeine arouses you by blocking the effects of adenosine, one of the substances that make you sleepy. That's why so many people use it to feel alert during the day. Alcohol suppresses parts of your central nervous system. Many people use it in the evening to help them relax, or even to sleep.

Although their effects are very different, both alcohol and caffeine can make it more difficult to get the sleep you need. Alcohol consumed before bedtime interferes with the quality of sleep, especially in the second half of the night. Mental and physical performance suffer the next day because of sleep loss, long after the alcohol itself has been metabolized and has worn off.

Consuming caffeine during the day also affects sleep, even if you had that last cup of coffee many hours before bed. Caffeine is a stimulant that promotes alertness by inhibiting chemicals in the brain that promote sleep.

In general, both alcohol and caffeine should be avoided in the hours before sleep. A cup of coffee after dinner might help you feel alert, but you'll likely still be feeling that way when your head is on your pillow. And a nightcap in the evening to help you sleep better will, in fact, have the opposite effect. The greater the number of hours between consuming either alcohol or caffeine and your bedtime, the better.

Researchers recently reviewed all previous studies and developed guidance on when caffeine intake should be cut off each day to avoid reducing time asleep at night. The general guidelines are as follows: A single cup of black tea generally contains too little caffeine to affect sleep. Your last cup of coffee (107 mg caffeine) should be approximately nine hours before bed. If you have an energy drink (217 mg caffeine), drink it more than 13 hours before your bedtime.

Cutting back on caffeine can be difficult. Caffeine withdrawal causes fatigue, which might entice you to have another cup of coffee. Stick with it, though, as fatigue will dissipate fairly quickly.

If you drink alcohol in the evening and your sleep is disrupted, especially in the second half of the night, the alcohol is a likely culprit. Try to cut back on the amount you consume and move it further away from bedtime.

At any time of day, consuming too much alcohol is unhealthy. The U.S. Department of Health and Human Services recommends limiting daily intake to two standard drinks for men and one drink for women. The National Institute on Alcohol Abuse and Alcoholism defines heavy drinking for men as four or more drinks on any day or 14 or more drinks per week, and for women as three or more drinks on any day or seven or more per week.

Nicotine

Nicotine is a stimulant, which can interfere with a good night's sleep. Nicotine also raises the risk of other health problems, such as cardiovascular disease and heart attack. Given the myriad negative health effects of this highly addictive chemical, quitting is by far the best path to take.

Technology has changed the way people consume nicotine, and vapes (e-cigarettes) have surged in popularity, especially among the young. Whichever way it's delivered, nicotine exerts a strong influence on sleep. Nicotine users are more likely to take longer to fall asleep, sleep less and have greater risk for insomnia. The more nicotine they consume, the worse they sleep. Also, people who use nicotine often do so at night, when its impact on sleep is greatest.

It can be hard to limit nicotine use to certain parts of the day in an effort to reduce its effects on sleep. Nicotine can prompt withdrawal symptoms within a few hours, creating an intense craving. When these cravings occur at night, they interfere with sleep, making it especially difficult to strategically limit nicotine. If you move up your last nicotine use during the day, it could be the withdrawal that hurts your sleep instead of the direct stimulation of the nicotine.

Quitting is an important step toward improving your sleep and your overall health. There are several safe and effective ways to quit nicotine that can be tailored to minimize withdrawal symptoms and sleep disturbances. Your doctor can help you find the best method.

Phones, tablets and televisions
Technology has opened up the world by providing us round-the-clock access to limitless streams of information and entertainment, all just by jabbing a finger at your handheld phone. It's also made it more difficult for many people to sleep. Websites and social media platforms are designed to keep you clicking, not to make you doze off. The content they offer can increase stress hormones, alter brain chemistry and put your body in a state of high arousal.

Electronic screens also emit a blue glow with particular potency for your eyes and brain. This blue light is especially good at resetting the body's internal clock (circadian rhythms). As part of a healthy nighttime routine, stop looking at screens an hour before bedtime. If an hour buffer isn't possible some nights, do your best to stop at least 30 minutes before you begin trying to sleep.

LED screens on televisions also emit light in the blue end of the spectrum. If possible, put the television somewhere other than your bedroom. This will help limit watching TV just before bed, when blue light is most damaging to sleep, and will also help train your body that your bedroom is a place for sleep.

Exercise
Exercise provides a number of benefits to your well-being, such as keeping your brain healthy, reducing the risk of heart disease, helping

control your weight and strengthening your bones and muscles. Exercise can also help you get a good night's sleep.

More than half the U.S. population doesn't get the recommended amount of exercise each week — a minimum of 150 minutes of moderately intense activity. You can fulfill exercise recommendations by doing any activity that gets your heart going, increases your breathing and works your muscles. For example, walking briskly for 30 minutes a day five days a week and doing muscle-strengthening activities two days a week will get you there.

For most people, exercise also reduces the time it takes to fall asleep and increases time spent in restorative deep sleep. And it works quickly, with a single session of exercise today helping you sleep better tonight. Keeping to a regular exercise routine has been shown to boost time spent asleep and overall quality of sleep.

There are no hard-and-fast rules about the right time to exercise. Your body and your schedule will be the most important factors influencing that. It may take trial and error to settle on a time that fits best into your routine and helps you sleep.

For some people, the best time to exercise might be after work. If that's the case for you, pay close attention to how nighttime exercise affects your sleep. It's a widely held belief that nighttime exercise and sleep don't mix. A late-night workout can rev up the body in a way that's not conducive to restfulness. However, research suggests that the body recovers fairly quickly.

Vigorous exercise one hour before bed can elevate your heart rate, change your body temperature and disrupt your sleep. In one study, participants who worked out an hour before bed took almost 15 minutes longer to fall asleep. Exercising two hours before bedtime, however, might provide enough of a gap for you. Intense exercise at least two hours before bed has been shown to help people fall asleep faster and sleep longer.

Naps

Like many people, shortly after lunch you may find your brain and body dragging, and what you wouldn't give for a nap! Naps can be an effective and efficient way to restore alertness, hit reset on your ability to concentrate and restore emotional resilience. But napping also can be counterproductive, leaving you feeling groggy and a bit disoriented, or making it harder for you to fall asleep at night.

So, should you nap, or shouldn't you? That depends on several factors, including how long you nap. Naps lasting a few minutes can be restorative, while long naps can leave you feeling sleepier when you wake than when you dozed off.

People have come to think of short, after-lunch rest periods as "power naps." The term was coined in the late 1990s to encourage

> **I KNOW THAT EXERCISE HELPS WITH SLEEP. SHOULD I WAKE UP EARLY TO FIT IN A WORKOUT, EVEN IF THAT MEANS I MIGHT GET LESS SLEEP?**
>
> Finding time in your day to exercise can be a challenge. Some people fit in time to exercise by sleeping less. People who work longer hours tend to exercise less than those who work shorter hours. Researchers also have found that people who exercise regularly in the morning before work sleep less, indicating that they may be setting their alarm clock earlier to fit in their workout.
>
> Perhaps this is an acceptable trade-off. If you feel alert and awake during the day after waking early to exercise, that could be a sign you've achieved a good balance between working out and sleeping. There's also reason to believe that morning exercise is better for most people, metabolically, in terms of curbing appetite and burning more calories.
>
> But if an early morning workout leaves you feeling sleepy, fatigued and perhaps moody during the day, this might not be the best approach.
>
> Sleep and exercise should go hand in hand as you develop healthy habits for your brain and body. Both require an investment of time, but the benefits are worth it. You may have to experiment to find what works best for you in your daily routine.

employers to allow short rest and sleep periods for their workers to boost performance. A key selling point was that they should be kept short.

A problem with long naps involves sleep inertia, the mental fog that can linger after you wake up. When you awaken from deep sleep, your brain can be muddled, your physical performance isn't what it could be, and you feel listless. Sleep inertia is much less common when waking up from the lighter stages of sleep. Ending a nap before you slip all the way into deep sleep can prevent sleep inertia and keep you from feeling groggy when you wake.

Short naps can be beneficial, boosting performance and making you feel alert when you wake up. They also can improve memory. Just as your brain works at night to store away memories for long-term retrieval, the same process can also occur during naps. Researchers have

---

I HAD TO STAY AWAKE ALL NIGHT FOR WORK. HOW DO I MAKE UP THAT SLEEP?

Try to get caught up as soon as possible, but recognize that you're not going to do it in one bout of sleep. If you need a little nap to make yourself functional, take a nap, but preferably not longer than 20 to 30 minutes so that you don't have horrible sleep inertia. Don't do anything that requires alertness for safety reasons until you've found time to enjoy a nice, long, uninterrupted sleep.

It could be two or three nights before you eventually get caught up. When you can arrange for a night of uninterrupted sleep, you should be fine. If you need to sleep a little longer the next couple of nights, that's OK.

If you find yourself staying awake all night regularly not because of work but because of insomnia, it's often best to power through. Avoiding a nap during the day will help you sleep better at night.

seen improvements in retention of learned facts and motor skills even after short, light naps.

One well-known study used something of a Goldilocks strategy, testing naps of different lengths — 5, 10, 20 or 30 minutes — to find the one that was just right. The benefits of the 5-minute nap wore off too soon. The 20- and 30-minute naps, which tended to include several minutes of deep sleep, left participants feeling groggy due to sleep inertia. The nap that was just right? The 10-minute nap, which led to improvements in alertness and performance immediately after waking that lasted for several hours.

If you're going to nap, do it right and keep it short. Naps of 30 minutes or less have a good chance of leaving you feeling restored and alert without the fogginess of sleep inertia.

There are some exceptions to the long nap rule. Longer napping after being deprived of sleep may help you feel and perform better. Long naps can also be essential for helping night shift workers stay alert and at peak performance on the job. Many athletes incorporate napping into their training and recovery routines, and these naps may be a bit longer. A recent review of the research on napping led one team of experts to conclude that naps can improve athletic performance. They recommended athletes limit naps to 20 to 90 minutes between 1 p.m. and 4 p.m.

If you sleep well at night and find a short nap during the day to be refreshing, then listen to your body and keep on napping. If, on the other hand, you generally sleep poorly, get fatigued and find yourself napping during the day to catch up on sleep, it could be that your naps are contributing to the problem instead of solving it.

Keep in mind that the need to nap also can be a signal that something else is wrong. Habitual napping has been associated with high blood pressure, depression, diabetes and cognitive decline, especially in older adults. If you find yourself needing more naps or being sleepy most days, discuss it with your doctor.

Relaxation techniques
Falling asleep comes more quickly when bedtime isn't abrupt but instead follows a few hours of winding down. For you, winding down might include structured relaxation activities or use of a meditation

app on your phone. (Don't use this as an excuse to check your social media accounts before bed!)

Relaxation is a complex interplay of physical and mental factors that you can guide and influence. Your body has a relaxation response, a physical state of deep rest that reduces your heart rate and lowers your blood pressure. Your mood and focus improve also.

Many people find relaxation techniques effective for enhancing the quality of their sleep as well as for helping establish a sense of calm and improving their overall well-being and mental health.

Here are three common relaxation techniques you can try tonight as part of your sleep routine:

- **Guided imagery.** Lying or sitting quietly, close your eyes and visualize a place or a situation you find peaceful and pleasant. Start adding details, tapping into as many of your senses as possible, including sight, hearing and touch. Put yourself in the place and explore it. Your body will begin to treat your experience as the real thing, allowing you to feel relaxed and calm, as if you were truly there.
- **Progressive muscle relaxation.** Systematically tensing and releasing the muscles in your body can be a slow, calming exercise. To give it a try, begin with your toes. Tense them for five seconds, then relax them for 30 seconds. Focus on the difference in sensations between tension and relaxation. Slowly move up your legs and the rest of your body, tensing and relaxing each muscle group until you reach your neck and head.
- **Deep breathing.** This therapy focuses on deep, relaxed breathing to reduce tension and stress. Find a comfortable position, sitting or lying down. Inhale slowly through your nose with your mouth closed and shoulders relaxed. Allow the air to fill your diaphragm. Pause for a second, then slowly release the air through your mouth. Repeat this cycle several times

In general, relaxation techniques haven't been studied well enough to determine how effectively they help people sleep. The American College of Physicians concluded that the evidence was insufficient to recommend relaxation techniques alone for insomnia. But it doesn't hurt to give them a try to see if they can help relax and calm you.

MANAGING WORRIES AND STRESS

Not everyone reacts to stress and worry in the same way. For some, worries can seem worse at night, keeping you awake as effectively as a loud noise or a bright light would. Your worries may seem untamable, coming and going into your consciousness as they please. In fact, there are several techniques you can use to put a leash on your worries and exert some command over them.

In some cases, it's the unfocused mind that allows worries to ramble, and focusing on them reins them in. Some people find scheduling worry time before bed to be helpful. While this might sound like a disagreeable way to spend a few minutes, it can have the effect of naming the things that float in and out of your head at night and putting them into a realistic perspective.

Other people find it cathartic to make a nightly list of the things they find worrisome. For each item, jot down a simple step that will help alleviate the worry. In some cases, that might even be "Think about it next week." You might find the list isn't as long as it may seem in the dark.

Other steps you can take include getting better organized and delegating some tasks to others. This not only helps manage the worry but also helps solve the problem causing it. Exercise can help alleviate worry and stress. Physical activity helps burn off stress-related tension. You might also consider taking a break from your normal routine and doing something enjoyable. And, of course, there's nothing like a good laugh to reduce or relieve tension.

The degree to which stress disrupts your sleep is known as sleep reactivity. High sleep reactivity is a recognized risk factor for insomnia. Some people who find themselves consumed with worry are diagnosed with generalized anxiety disorder, which is a treatable condition. If you find that worry and stress are harming your sleep or sense of well-being, discuss it with your doctor.

SAVING YOUR BEDROOM FOR SLEEP

Your bedroom may be a bit of a multipurpose room, the place where you watch television, have your home office, or sit and read. To help you sleep, it's important to establish your bedroom as a place for sleep and little else. If possible, use your bed only for sleep and sex. If you have the space, move the television or your work desk to another room. When you enter the bedroom at bedtime, it should signal to your body that it's time for sleep.

Some experts say you should make your bedroom like a tomb — dark, silent and cool. While you might think that sounds a little spooky, the more you can foster a sense of calm and quiet, the better your chances of creating the right conditions for restorative sleep. Here are some things to consider as you create the ideal environment.

SEX AND SLEEP

Many people find that they sleep better after sexual activity and orgasm. Sex and orgasm prompt the internal release of oxytocin and prolactin, hormones that reduce stress, foster a sense of calm and improve sleep. Sex also reduces cortisol, the so-called stress hormone that can often be the enemy of sleep. Research indicates that prolactin release is up to four times greater in sex with a partner than with masturbation.

Perceptions about the sleep benefits of sex vary widely. In one survey, most people found that sex with a partner helped them fall asleep and improved their sleep quality. This was more likely to be true for men than for women.

Some people, however, find that sexual activity leaves them feeling less sleepy. Surprisingly few studies have been done on the impact of sex on sleep. Nevertheless, some experts believe that for some individuals, sexual activity can be a useful part of a sleep routine.

Dark vs. light

Most people find it easier to sleep in the dark, without the brain-stimulating effects of light. Deciding how light should be incorporated into your healthy sleep habits is more complicated than just turning off the bedside lamp. Your body is constantly making adjustments based on how much light it's exposed to around the clock.

Although we take it for granted, the ability to turn darkness into light with a flip of the switch has a profound effect on the human body. Your eyes don't only allow you to see; they also pick up cues about what time of day it is just by sensing light. This influences your body's internal clock and all the things that obey it, from your physical and mental performance to your need for sleep.

As part of your effort to improve your sleep habits, make your bedroom as dark as possible and try to expose yourself to bright light during the day, especially in the morning.

Much is made of the ability of blue light, including the kind emitted from the screens of electronic devices, to upset your circadian rhythm. While light in other parts of the spectrum isn't as potent, it too has an effect on your body's clockwork. Even with your eyes closed as you sleep, light in your room at night has a measurable impact on your circadian rhythm by shifting the release of hormones associated with sleep.

Researchers have identified other health effects from nighttime light. In one study, involving over 43,000 women, the researchers found that those who slept with a light or television on in their room were more likely to be obese and continue to gain weight. A small night-light in the room didn't produce the same result.

To help your body prepare for sleep, begin to reduce light levels in your home three hours before bedtime. In bedrooms and areas where you spend a lot of time in the evening, it can also be beneficial to install light bulbs that give off light that's warmer in color, labeled 2,700K to 3,000K.

For the best sleep, make your bedroom as dark as possible. In some places, especially cities, this might require opaque window shades. Some people find eye masks effective in reducing light. They can be especially helpful for shift workers who must sleep during the day or where blackout curtains aren't available. If you're likely to get up during the night and are at risk of falling in a darkened room, use a low-intensity night-light.

In the morning, embrace the light. Do your best to expose yourself to bright light for at least a few hours early in the day. Exposure to bright light after you wake keeps your circadian rhythm in sync and helps you fall asleep faster at night and feel less sleepy during the day.

Quiet vs. noise
Your sleeping body responds to a noise in the night as if it were a potential danger. Your heart rate increases, blood pressure rises and adrenaline flows. You may stir, even if you don't wake up.

Nighttime noise fragments sleep, leaving you feeling less restored and altering your stages of sleep. Sounds can reduce slow-wave and rapid eye movement (REM) sleep, while increasing the lightest stage of sleep. By one estimate, nearly 42 million Americans have their sleep disturbed due to noise from automobiles, trucks and airplanes. While we may believe that we can learn to live with the noise, our bodies never truly get used to it. People who are subjected to airplane noise, for example, are aroused or awakened even after exposure over an extended time.

Do your best to make your bedroom a quiet place at night. In some cases, this may require asking others in the house to change their behavior, perhaps turning down music or a television. Improving acoustics can make it easier to get good sleep. In some homes, noise can be tempered with sound-reducing curtains, rugs or carpets, or even acoustic panels.

Rather than strive for silence, some people opt to block out the sound. The American Academy of Sleep Medicine recommends trying white noise if nighttime sounds disturb your sleep.

White noise is made up of all the frequencies we hear. Any sound that's added to it, such as noises from the street, is masked. Some people find that when they use white noise, they're no longer awakened by outside sounds. Studies of residents in noisy areas in New York City found that white noise helped people fall asleep faster and sleep longer. If quiet is unattainable in your home, consider trying a white noise device.

Earplugs are also a simple and inexpensive remedy for many people. Both earplugs and eye masks have proven beneficial to patients in intensive care units, where round-the-clock noise and light can make sleep difficult.

Cool vs. warm

Yet another way your body runs in time with circadian rhythms is by way of your internal thermostat, which gets dialed up and down over the course of a 24-hour day. You reach your lowest body temperature at about 4 a.m. It then begins to rise as the time to wake up nears.

Temperature — both inside your body and in the environment around you — plays an important role in sleep. A room that is either too cold or too warm can interfere with the quality of sleep. Research

---

DOES WHAT YOU WEAR AFFECT YOUR SLEEP?

Of all the things in your nighttime environment, none is closer to you than your clothes. Your choice of what you wear to bed, including the kind of fabric it's made of, can play a significant role in your sleep.

Controlling temperature and airflow is important, and it can be increasingly difficult for your body to maintain a cool temperature as you age.

In warmer temperatures, cotton can be a better choice than polyester. Cotton wicks moisture away from the body more efficiently than polyester does, keeping you cooler. Cotton absorbs 24% of its weight in moisture, polyester, less than 1%. Wool is even more absorbent, at 35%, though wool sleepwear isn't as common as other types in the United States, and you may not like its feel.

Above all, consider function over style, and place a priority on the garment not binding or bunching, which could wake you up. Some people choose not to wear any sleepwear at all. Sleeping naked for some is the best way to keep cool and sleep well.

In search of quality sleep

shows that people wake more often and have less restorative deep sleep and REM sleep in rooms that are too warm or too cold.

Make your bedroom as cool as you can and still be comfortable. An ideal temperature for sleep is between 64 F and 68 F or even a few degrees lower. The actual temperature of your room will be a matter of personal preference.

Most people also use sleepwear, sheets and blankets to adjust the temperature immediately around them, creating a personal microclimate. This can help partners with different preferences achieve the temperature that suits their own sleep needs best.

Maintaining optimal temperature often requires heating in the winter and air-conditioning in the summer, which can be costly. If reducing your bedroom temperature isn't possible or is too expensive, using a fan may work. Moving air over your skin can help cool you and reduce the number of times you wake. Research has found that instead of keeping you awake, the sensation of moving air helps create a monotonous feeling that encourages sleep.

Taking a bath within an hour or two of sleep also has been shown to help regulate body temperature and decrease the time it takes to fall asleep.

Alarm clocks

Most of us wake up to an alarm clock. In general, using an alarm probably means that you're not getting as much sleep as you would without it. But all of us function with a little bit less sleep than we might otherwise get.

If you're feeling well rested and are getting seven hours of sleep or close to it, you're probably not sleep-deprived. You're just trying to get to work on time.

If, however, you're always waking up with an alarm — and especially if you experience sleepiness later in the day — you probably are sleep-deprived. If you can't set the alarm later, then you should consider making your bedtime earlier.

Hitting the snooze
In 1956, General Electric-Telechron released the Snooz-Alarm, and for the first time, sleepers were tempted to hit a button allowing them to

stay in bed just a few more minutes. Followed by a few more. And maybe just a few more!

Since then, the snooze button and its electronic descendants have become a regular part of the morning routines for millions of people. Studies indicate that most people who use alarms, the vast majority of U.S. adults, also use the snooze feature.

Ultimately, though, snooze alarms are only making it harder to wake up and feel refreshed and alert. They lengthen sleep inertia, that disoriented, foggy and sometimes stumbling state between sleep and waking. Usually sleep inertia fades 15 to 30 minutes after waking, but snooze alarms may extend it.

In one study, a survey of Japanese college students found that nearly three-fourths of those who woke to an alarm used a snooze feature. Most hit snooze four or five times each morning, at five-minute intervals over about 20 minutes or more. After monitoring the students as they woke, the researchers concluded that use of the snooze feature increased sleep inertia and fatigue.

If you're in the habit of hitting the snooze button, try weaning yourself from it. Use music as your alarm. Open the curtains or turn on the lights to make the room as bright as possible. You might need to put your alarm across the room. Getting out of bed when the alarm goes off may help wake you enough to keep you from snoozing.

If you typically burn 20 minutes hitting the snooze button, set your alarm 20 minutes later. The urgency to get to work or school on time may help motivate you, and you may get a few more minutes of sleep.

Alarm clocks on weekends

We all catch up a little on sleep on the weekends. Some extra sleep may make the rest of your week and the quality of your sleep better. If you sleep in, however, try to keep it under one hour, if possible.

Also, try not to make sleeping in on weekends a habit, or a way to make up for lost sleep during the week. Because regularity is important to good sleep, you also don't want a wide discrepancy between weekdays and weekends. Sleeping in on weekend mornings could start interfering with your ability to fall asleep on Sunday night.

Maintaining a sleep schedule is important for overall good sleep. If setting an alarm on the weekend helps you to sleep better through the week, then do so. But it's also OK if on weekends you set the alarm to go off a bit later — but no more than an hour.

Your bed

By adopting good habits, you can make your bed into a place your body associates with sleep. To get there, though, the bed first has to be a place your body associates with comfort.

A poor mattress can make it difficult to sleep and can even leave you with aches, including back pain, throughout the day. Test your current mattress as if you were in a store shopping for a new one. If it's not comfortable enough to support a good night's sleep and not one you'd buy today, consider investing in a replacement.

Some research suggests that a medium-firm mattress is best for comfort and optimal alignment of the spine, which should remain as

---

WEIGHTED BLANKETS

While many people seek out the lightest blankets possible so as not to disturb them during sleep, others go in the opposite direction, piling on blankets that can weigh upward of 30 pounds. In theory, the heft of these weighted blankets creates a soothing, calming feeling by mimicking human touch.

Weighted blankets may be loaded with metal chains or with beads made from a variety of materials. Some are handwoven from heavy cords. They can be expensive, with prices ranging up to several hundred dollars.

Studies suggest that weighted blankets may help some people sleep. In one noteworthy study of people with psychiatric disorders, using a weighted blanket improved sleep, increased daily activity and reduced fatigue and anxiety.

While the medical literature suggests that weighted blankets may decrease anxiety, there's not enough evidence that they help alleviate insomnia to recommend them.

straight during sleep as when you are standing. Medium-firm mattresses have been shown to improve sleep quality for people with lower back pain. Ultimately, mattress choices are intensely personal and highly individual. Some people find that a mattress with adjustable firmness suits them best.

The ability of the mattress surface to keep you cool can also be a factor. Whether you feel warm or cool as you lie atop the mattress can affect how well you sleep. Manufacturers claim some mattress pads are made of cooling foam, and devices are available that circulate chilled air or water through a mattress pad. While science has clearly established that cooler temperatures are good for sleep, there's little research to back up claims that the pads improve sleep. A small pilot study of women 45 to 59 years old found that a water-containing cooling mattress pad significantly reduced the women's hot flashes and improved their sleep. These devices can be expensive, and some require cleaning and other maintenance.

Pets in bed

Many people derive tremendous emotional benefit from the cat or dog that shares their home — and often their bed. For some, one of those benefits might be a better night's sleep.

For many others, however, a pet can make good sleep difficult. Your pets' internal clocks are different from yours, so they naturally have times when they're alert and you need to be asleep. Many pets also tend not to observe boundaries wishfully delineated as "their part of the bed." At night, even a small dog can suddenly seem to have very long legs.

To get all the lifetime benefits that sleeping well brings, reconsider your pets' sleeping arrangements if they share the bed with you. Uninterrupted sleep might need to take priority over the satisfaction you and your pet get from sleeping in the same bed.

Here's a list of factors, developed by Mayo Clinic, to consider as you sort through this complex and potentially emotional issue:
- How well do you sleep?
- How well does your human bed partner sleep?
- Does either of you have pet allergies?
- How big is the bedroom? The bed?

- Does the pet sleep soundly?
- Is the pet quiet?
- How many pets are there on the bed?
- Where on the bed does the pet sleep?
- Is it possible to exclude the pet from the bedroom?
- Does the pet require your attention at night because of needs such as going to the bathroom or taking medications?
- Does the pet enhance your sense of security?
- Does having the pet in your bed help you relax?

If you're sleeping fine with your pet, there may be no need to make a change. If your sleep is poor, though, consider trying different arrangements to discover if it improves. Breaking your pet's habit of sharing your bed might take a few nights, prompting some whining, barking or meowing. However, the potential long-term benefit to your sleep and health could be significant.

5

Do you have a sleep disorder?

A sleep disorder is sometimes defined as a disturbance of normal sleep patterns that negatively affects your daily life. To you, such a simple description may seem to fall far short of the disruption to your health and well-being that your sleep problems are causing.

As you may know only too well, a sleep disorder can take a toll on your mood and thinking, your performance at work, your relationship with your partner and your quality of life. It can leave you more likely to make mistakes, or even fall asleep doing something that requires your full attention — including driving a car. Too little sleep also can put you at greater risk for other serious, potentially life-changing health conditions.

A sleep disorder is likely to leave you in one of two extreme states: intensely sleepy or frustratingly sleepless. In the short term, you may try to bear with these symptoms and manage them as best you can. But if they continue for an extended period, it's likely time to seek medical help.

There may be other indications, too, that you have a condition that's robbing you of the benefits of good sleep. You may experience unusual breathing patterns or bothersome movements while sleeping or be plagued by an uncomfortable urge to move your legs when trying to sleep. You also may do unusual things during sleep, such as get up and walk or eat. Or your sleep schedule may be highly irregular. Any one of these can be a sign of a sleep problem that should be addressed.

In this chapter, we briefly introduce you to some of the most common sleep disorders so that you can better understand what may be causing problems for you or a loved one. (These conditions are discussed in depth in later chapters.) We'll also give you a sense of when you might consider making an appointment with a doctor and what a medical professional may need to know to identify and treat your problem.

Perhaps you've tried fixing your sleep problems on your own with some of the lifestyle changes discussed in prior chapters. If these steps haven't helped much and you're still excessively sleepy or exasperatingly sleepless, your doctor's office should be your next stop.

The good news is that most sleep disorders can be successfully treated to reduce or eliminate their symptoms, putting you on a path to reclaim the benefits that a good night's sleep provides.

For many disorders, treatment often begins by establishing good sleep habits, including developing a sleep routine and making healthy choices about what you eat and drink. Other steps may include specific therapies intended to reduce or eliminate your symptoms. Some can be life-changing.

In addition to helping determine if you have a sleep condition, the purpose of this chapter is to provide a deeper understanding of what you can expect from your healthcare team as they address your sleep concerns.

RED FLAGS

Sleeplessness or sleepiness isn't always a sure sign of a sleep disorder. Everyone has times when they can't get to sleep, or they feel unusually tired during the day. Alcohol and caffeine can make it difficult to get quality sleep, and their effects can even mimic those of a sleep disorder. Plus, as you age, a good night's sleep can become more elusive.

Many sleep problems are short-lived and tied to stressful life events. Though troublesome, they can often be overcome by sticking with good sleep habits. Sometimes, though, the problem becomes more persistent and develops into a sleep disorder. How do you know if what you're experiencing is typical or if you have a problem?

In the broadest sense, the red flags for a sleep disorder are regularly having trouble falling or staying asleep or being excessively tired during the day. If these symptoms are affecting your daily performance and persist for an extended period, there's reason to be concerned.

The following list was compiled by the National Institutes of Health. If any of these items describe ongoing problems you or your partner is experiencing, discuss it with your doctor.

- It regularly takes you more than 30 minutes to fall asleep when you're tired.
- You wake up many times during the night and have trouble falling back asleep.
- You wake up too early in the morning.
- You feel sleepy during the day, take frequent naps or fall asleep while doing other things.
- Your bed partner hears you snore or make other sounds in your sleep, including snorts, gasps or choking noises.
- Your partner notices that you stop breathing for short periods during sleep.
- You have sensations in your legs that are hard to describe but may feel like creeping, tingling or crawling.
- Your partner notices that your legs or arms make sudden jerking movements frequently during sleep.
- You have episodes of sudden muscle weakness when you are angry or fearful.
- Sometimes you wake but feel you cannot move.

In some cases, these signs and symptoms might indicate not a sleep disorder but a different medical condition. It's important to determine the cause of your problem so that you can work together with your doctor to effectively treat it.

COMMON SLEEP DISORDERS

Countless people are afflicted by sleep problems. If you believe you could be one of them, you have plenty of company. One oft-cited statistic estimates that more than 50 million adults in the United States have a sleep disorder, though the number could well be much higher.

A few conditions account for most sleep disorders. Though the most obvious outward signs — sleepiness or sleeplessness — can result from nearly any one of them, each has a different cause and treatment. For some conditions you may need to see a specialist. We discuss many of these disorders in greater detail in later chapters.

Insomnia
Trouble falling or staying asleep — insomnia — is both a symptom and a medical disorder. Many people occasionally have insomnia symptoms, with about one-third of U.S. adults reporting trouble sleeping. For many, insomnia arrives each night in an anxious expanse of minutes or hours after bedtime when sleep remains elusive. For others, insomnia may take the form of waking up several hours too early and being unable to fall back asleep. Occasionally, insomnia can be accompanied by excessive daytime sleepiness or fatigue, which can interfere with work and other activities.

Often, insomnia-related signs and symptoms are short-lived, lasting days, weeks or perhaps a couple of months. This is considered acute insomnia disorder. Eventually, as stressful situations are resolved, sleep difficulties diminish with time. Good sleep habits and coping skills also can help limit the impact and duration of the problem.

Sometimes, though, insomnia symptoms persist, and in some cases develop into a lasting disorder. When signs and symptoms of insomnia last for more than three months, it's considered chronic insomnia disorder.

Insomnia may appear on its own or it may be connected to another condition that's making it difficult for you to fall asleep. Insomnia can emerge with a sleep disorder such as sleep apnea, or it can appear in tandem with other physical or mental conditions, such as pain or depression.

In some cases, difficulty falling or staying asleep isn't insomnia at all but the effects of another problem or condition, such as certain medications, substance abuse or an undiagnosed disease. Your doctor will sort through your health history and lifestyle habits to help arrive at a diagnosis. Though your symptoms can seem dire, insomnia is highly treatable.

Sleep apnea

The word *apnea* means "to stop breathing." Sleep apnea is characterized by numerous short interruptions or other abnormalities in breathing during the night. It's estimated that 25 million U.S. adults have the condition.

Snoring is a common sign of sleep apnea. Interruptions in breathing associated with the disorder also can result in unusual noises, such as snorting or gasping. The condition is considered mild if you experience an average of 5 to 15 abnormal breathing events per hour through the night. Moderate disease is defined by 15 to 30 disruptions per hour, and severe disease by more than 30 disruptions an hour during sleep.

Sleep apnea takes several forms, each with unique underlying causes. Obstructive sleep apnea is the most common and is characterized by intermittent collapse and blockage of your upper airway, which produces symptoms such as snoring, snorting and gasping. The condition is most common in people who are overweight, have certain physical upper airway or jaw characteristics, or have a family history of sleep apnea. Sleep apnea also can appear along with certain medical conditions such as cardiovascular disease, hypothyroidism and diabetes.

Another form of sleep apnea, called central sleep apnea, is less common and involves a breakdown in signaling from the brain that interrupts breathing. Central sleep apnea is most often encountered in individuals with heart disease.

Left untreated, sleep apnea decreases your quality of life and increases your risk of cardiovascular disease, stroke and death.

Restless legs syndrome

Also known as RLS, restless legs syndrome causes an uncomfortable sensation and urge to move your legs. This can make it difficult or impossible to fall asleep. People with mild RLS may experience these urges a few times a month, while individuals whose condition is more severe may feel them nightly. Relief may come after moving your legs around, rubbing them together, massaging them, or getting up and walking.

By some estimates, up to 10% of U.S. adults have RLS, and the condition is more common among women than men. Children, too, can be affected by RLS, though it becomes more common with age. When the condition begins before age 45, it's known as early-onset RLS, and it typically progresses slowly. Late-onset RLS begins after age 45 and often worsens quickly.

The causes of restless legs syndrome remain unclear, though researchers have identified some genetic and environmental factors that may contribute to it. It may be associated with abnormalities in levels of dopamine, a brain neurotransmitter, or low levels of iron. Some treatments include medications or supplements to correct the levels. Symptoms also may be made worse by caffeine, alcohol or nicotine.

Narcolepsy

Narcolepsy is characterized by extreme sleepiness during the day (hypersomnia) that can lead to struggles staying awake, including nodding off suddenly without warning. Narcolepsy may cause you to fall asleep in the middle of an activity, including eating, working or driving. It can also include frequent waking in the night. Other symptoms may include sudden, brief muscle weakness associated with strong emotions (cataplexy), a sense of paralysis when falling asleep or waking, and vivid hallucinations when waking or falling asleep.

The condition most often begins in adolescence and affects about 1 in 2,000 people in the United States.

Circadian rhythm disorders

Circadian rhythm disorders, also known as sleep-wake cycle disorders, are problems that occur when your body's internal clock — which tells you when it's time to sleep or wake — is out of sync with your environment. As a result, you're unable to sleep well and be fully awake at the right time.

Sleep-wake cycle disorders may have a direct cause, such as frequent overseas travel and jet lag or a job that requires working the night shift. In some cases, there may be no clear trigger for disorganized sleep-wake cycles.

One disorder that fits into this category is delayed sleep-wake phase disorder. With this condition, the time you feel sleepy and can fall asleep and the time you feel rested enough to wake up arrive much later than what's typical or what you desire. Delayed sleep-wake phase disorder often leads to a loss of sleep and an inability to wake up, and is frequently accompanied by depression. The condition is most prevalent among adolescents and is more severe than simply staying up late, common among teens.

About one-third of people who work evenings or nights show signs of a circadian rhythm disorder due to shift work. Because they're out of sync with their internal clocks, their body is telling them to sleep when they need to work, and they feel alert when they finally have time for sleep. In addition to getting too little sleep, their sleep is often of poor quality.

Sleepwalking and other parasomnias
Sleepwalking (somnambulism) is the best-known form of parasomnia, a condition in which someone acts in unusual and undesirable ways during sleep. People who are sleepwalking can look as if they're awake, though they may have a blank expression. Sleepwalking episodes can last a few seconds or up to a half hour and can involve complex activities such as getting dressed or going to the bathroom. In rare cases, a person who is sleepwalking will leave home. Sleepwalking and some other forms of parasomnia are most common between the ages of 5 and 25.

Other parasomnias include talking or eating during sleep. A sleep-related eating disorder is characterized by sleepwalking that includes binge eating. It often involves consumption of high-calorie foods, but it can include things that are inappropriate to eat, such as uncooked meat. In some cases, the person doesn't remember doing these things and might be told about it by others or see the evidence the next morning.

Sleep terrors, another parasomnia, can involve screaming and a look of intense fear. Someone having a sleep terror may get out of bed and try to run. These episodes usually last a few minutes or less. They're most often seen in children, even as young as preschool age. Though it's rare, adults can experience such episodes as well.

WHEN TO SEE A DOCTOR

If sleepiness, sleeplessness or unusual behaviors during sleep are interfering with your work, health or quality of life, discuss it with your primary care provider. That conversation, and possibly some subsequent tests and appointments, can lead to answers about the cause of your condition and how to treat it.

The first step in arriving at a diagnosis is generally to obtain a thorough sleep history, getting to know all about your sleep patterns and

EXPLODING HEAD SYNDROME

It hopefully comes as no surprise that this rare and poorly named condition doesn't involve an actual explosion of the head. Rather, the syndrome is a condition in which a person is woken by what sounds like a loud bang, a noise as intense as a nearby thunderclap or a bomb going off. However, no such noise occurred.

Symptoms include:
- Waking suddenly to the noise of an explosion in your head.
- Being frightened when you wake.
- Having no feelings of pain.

The condition can appear in children as young as age 10, but the average age when it first occurs is 58. The perceived loud sound may be related to another sleep disorder, a medical condition or a mental health disorder.

environment and the concerns you have. Some questions your doctor might ask include:
- What do you do in the evening before going to bed?
- What time do you go to bed?
- How long does it take you to fall asleep?
- Are you interrupted during sleep?
- Do you wake up on your own or to an alarm?
- If you use an alarm, what time does it go off, and do you believe you are spending enough time in bed?
- Do you feel sleepy when waking up or during the day?
- Do you ever nod off at work or in social situations?
- Do you nap?

Also be prepared to discuss your medications, as well as use of caffeine, alcohol, nicotine, cannabis and other substances.

It may help to share with your doctor what a typical night is like for you, highlighting the sleep-related problems you're experiencing. If you sleep with a partner, use that person as a sounding board for the information you want to pass along to your doctor. Your partner might have additional information, having seen — and possibly heard — you while you're asleep. If you disrupt your partner's sleep during the night, it can be helpful to bring that person with you to the appointment.

If you use an app that records your sleep patterns, bring along a printout of some recent results. Your doctor may wish to look at it. While the information isn't accurate enough to be used as the basis for a diagnosis, it may provide some general indications about your sleep patterns that your doctor finds useful.

DIAGNOSING SLEEP DISORDERS

Doctors use several tools to help get to the root cause of a sleep disorder. At your visit, your doctor may ask you to fill out a questionnaire about your sleep patterns and habits and the quality of your sleep. Your doctor may also perform a physical examination and have you undergo some tests.

Sleep questionnaires
In determining if you have a sleep disorder, and which type, you may be asked to complete one or more of the following questionnaires.

The STOP-Bang or Berlin apnea questionnaire
If you or your doctor suspects you have sleep apnea, you might be asked specific questions as part of a questionnaire with an intriguing name: STOP-Bang. It can help estimate your risk of having obstructive sleep apnea, and perhaps even gauge its severity. STOP-Bang is an acronym, with each letter serving as a prompt for one of eight questions. Four of the questions are self-reportable facts about your sleep or health, and four provide demographic information.

The questions cover whether you snore, are tired during the day or have been observed not breathing during sleep. You're also asked your age and sex, the size of your shirt collar, your body mass index and if you have high blood pressure. Your answers will help your doctor determine your risk of obstructive sleep apnea as low, intermediate or high.

The results of the evaluation are just one component in making a diagnosis. For diagnosing obstructive sleep apnea, the American Academy of Sleep Medicine recommends that questionnaire results be combined with a sleep history, a physical examination, and a sleep study (polysomnography) or home sleep apnea test.

Insomnia Severity Index
With seven questions that take about a minute to answer, the Insomnia Severity Index questionnaire can help determine the difference between mild and serious insomnia disorder. The questionnaire may first be used as a screening tool and then used again during treatment to gauge progress.

The questionnaire's focus is on the last two weeks, probing your level of difficulty falling asleep and staying asleep, and whether you feel that you wake up too early. It asks how satisfied you are with your sleep and whether your sleep problems interfere with your daily life, your memory or your mood. Other questions include whether your sleep problems are noticeable to others and how distressed you are about them.

INSOMNIA SEVERITY INDEX (ISI)

Name: _____ Date: _____

1. Please rate the current (i.e., last 2 weeks) **SEVERITY** of your insomnia problem(s).

	None	Mild	Moderate	Severe	Very
Difficulty falling asleep	0	1	2	3	4
Difficulty staying asleep	0	1	2	3	4
Problem waking up too early	0	1	2	3	4

2. How **SATISFIED**/dissatisfied are you with your current sleep pattern?

Very Satisfied				Very Dissatisfied
0	1	2	3	4

3. To what extent do you consider your sleep problem to **INTERFERE** with your daily functioning (e.g., daytime fatigue, ability to function at work/daily chores, concentration, memory, mood, etc.)?

Not at All Interfering	A Little	Somewhat	Much	Very Much Interfering
0	1	2	3	4

4. How **NOTICEABLE** to others do you think your sleeping problem is in terms of impairing the quality of your life?

Not at All Noticeable	Barely	Somewhat	Much	Very Much Noticeable
0	1	2	3	4

5. How **WORRIED**/distressed are you about your current sleep problem?

Not at All	A Little	Somewhat	Much	Very Much
0	1	2	3	4

Guidelines for Scoring/Interpretation:
Add scores for all seven items (1a + 1b + 1c + 2 + 3 + 4 + 5)
Total score ranges from 0 to 28
- 0-7 = No clinically significant insomnia
- 8-14 = Subthreshold insomnia
- 15-21 = Clinical insomnia (moderate severity)
- 22-28 = Clinical insomnia (severe)

Copyright © 2001 Bastien et al. Reprinted with permission.

The U.S. Department of Veterans Affairs has a version of the questionnaire that you can take online and immediately get an assessment, which ranges from "no clinically significant insomnia" to "clinical insomnia (severe)."

Pittsburgh Sleep Quality Index
This questionnaire was developed in the 1980s to help differentiate "good" sleepers from "poor" ones. It uses 19 questions to arrive at a score of sleep quality. The questionnaire can help pinpoint symptoms of insomnia, but it also covers broader issues of sleep quality.

This questionnaire is often used in research and is sometimes used to help physicians understand how well someone is sleeping.

Epworth Sleepiness Scale
The Epworth Sleepiness Scale is a practical, though not highly precise, way to quantify how tired you feel and how drowsiness affects your life. It asks you to rate the likelihood that you would nod off while doing various activities, including reading, watching TV, lying down to rest, and talking to someone, or sitting in stopped traffic.

Excessive daytime sleepiness can be a symptom of many disorders, including obstructive sleep apnea, insomnia or narcolepsy. If you or your doctor is concerned about your daytime sleepiness, you might be given this short questionnaire. However, it's not widely used as a screening tool to determine if a sleep study is appropriate.

International Restless Legs Severity Scale
If you have symptoms of restless legs syndrome, a questionnaire can help determine its severity. The International Restless Legs Severity Scale questionnaire comes in two forms, one given by your doctor and one that you can take yourself. Both measure the intensity and frequency of your physical symptoms, as well as the sleep problems they cause.

You're asked to rate the severity of discomfort in your legs and arms and the need to move around, as well as how much relief that movement brings. You also indicate how often you have symptoms and how much they affect your sleep, your life and your mood.

EPWORTH SLEEPINESS SCALE

How likely are you to nod off or fall asleep in the following situations, in contrast to feeling just tired? This refers to your usual way of life in recent times.

Even if you haven't done some of these things recently, try to work out how they would have affected you. It is important that you answer each question as best you can.

Use the following scale to choose the most appropriate number for each situation.

	Would never nod off 0	Slight chance of nodding off 1	Moderate chance of nodding off 2	High chance of nodding off 3
Sitting and reading				
Watching TV				
Sitting, inactive, in a public place (e.g., in a meeting, theater, or dinner event)				
As a passenger in a car for an hour or more without stopping for a break				
Lying down to rest when circumstances permit				
Sitting quietly after a meal without alcohol				
In a car, while stopped for a few minutes in traffic or at a light				

Add up your points to get your total score. A score of 10 or greater raises concern: you may need to get more sleep, improve your sleep practices, or seek medical attention to determine why you are sleepy.

© 1990-1997 MW Johns. Reprinted with permission.

Do you have a sleep disorder?

Sleep diary

You may be asked to keep a sleep diary to help identify your sleep patterns and reveal any underlying problems. A sleep diary often comes in the form of a grid that you fill out in the morning and evening. It should be completed for at least seven consecutive days, including weekends, to be most accurate. You may be asked to keep a diary for two full weeks.

One version, available online as a free download from the U.S. National Heart, Lung, and Blood Institute, has one section to be filled out before going to bed and another to be completed in the morning. In the evening, it asks you to record how many caffeinated and alcoholic drinks you had and when, the number and length of any naps, how much exercise you got and how sleepy you felt during the day. In the morning, it asks you to log the time you went to bed and got out of bed, the number of times you awoke, how long it took you to fall asleep, medicines you took and how alert you felt when you got up.

Sleep study

A sleep study, known medically as polysomnography, is a wide-ranging test of your brain and body during sleep that records and compiles readings from several different types of sensors attached to your skin. The combined data provides your doctor a complete picture of the biological functioning (physiology) of your sleep through an entire night. This test, conducted in a sleep clinic, is considered the gold standard. It can be helpful in diagnosing sleep apnea or as part of a series of tests to diagnose narcolepsy and other sleep disorders.

The study is overseen by a technician who attaches the equipment and monitors the test through the night. Electrodes are placed in specific spots around your head with a special adhesive, or in some cases with an elastic cap. They measure brain waves that indicate the different stages of sleep. Sensors are secured near your right and left eyes to track the motion that indicates rapid eye movement (REM) sleep and the slow eye-rolling movements of drowsiness. Electrodes also are used to measure muscle activity in the leg and chin to detect movement during REM sleep.

Belts around your body and airflow sensors gather information on breathing. A pulse oximeter measures your heartbeat and how well your body is absorbing and using oxygen. Sometimes microphones and cameras are used to pick up snoring or other sounds and to capture unusual body movements or positions.

While a sleep study is often used as a diagnostic tool for sleep apnea, it also can be helpful in developing or monitoring treatment plans.

Home sleep apnea test
Technological advances have made it possible to gather many of the measurements included in a sleep study at home. A home sleep apnea test generally is less costly and more convenient than a full sleep apnea study conducted in a sleep center. For individuals with signs and symptoms indicating obstructive sleep apnea, this test can accurately identify the condition 90% of the time. Because the test is designed specifically for sleep apnea, it's not typically used to diagnose other sleep disorders.

POLYSOMNOGRAPHY

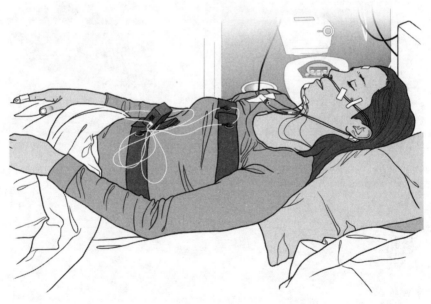

This study is done in a sleep clinic. You're attached to equipment that monitors your heart, lung and brain activity, breathing patterns, arm and leg movements, and blood oxygen levels while you sleep.

Home sleep apnea tests measure several different functions, though devices vary. Measurements may include the amount of effort required to breathe, the amount of airflow through your nose, whether you snore, oxygen levels in your blood, your heart rate and your body movements. Some devices track peripheral arterial tone, a noninvasive measure of the blood vessels in your fingertips that can help gauge the frequency of breathing problems and estimate the presence of different sleep stages. A home test doesn't include a recording of brain activity (electroencephalogram, or EEG), which accurately reveals how much time is spent in each stage of sleep.

The technology used in home sleep apnea tests continues to evolve, and the devices are continuously becoming more convenient and user-friendly. The Food and Drug Administration (FDA) has

HOME SLEEP APNEA TESTS

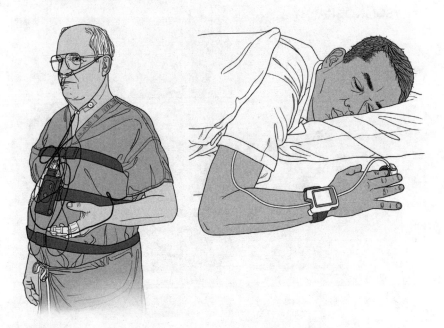

Home sleep apnea tests measure your heart rate, blood oxygen level, air flow and breathing patterns. Newer models, as shown at right, are easier to use.

WHAT TO EXPECT WITH A HOME SLEEP APNEA TEST

A home sleep apnea test is a relatively easy, noninvasive way for your doctor to record and measure how well you're breathing through the night while sleeping in your own bed.

Here's what you can expect on the day of your home sleep apnea study. Typically, you'll be asked to follow a checklist of dos and don'ts. The checklist may include the following:

- *Do* read and follow all instructions that come with the test.
- *Don't* drink coffee, tea, soda or anything else with caffeine after noon.
- *Do* consume your normal amount of alcohol, unless your physician tells you not to.
- *Do* eat your normal meals, but *don't* eat dinner too close to bedtime.
- *Don't* nap.
- *Don't* use heavy amounts of hairstyling products, makeup or body creams, which can interfere with the sensors.
- If a finger probe will be used to measure oxygen levels, *do* remove any acrylic nails and nail polish.
- *Do* take all your medications, unless your physician tells you not to.
- *Do* stick to your normal routine while preparing for bed.
- *Do* go to bed and wake up at the usual time.
- *Do* write down your sleep routine.

When waking in the morning, turn off the device and remove the sensors according to instructions. Return the device, if required.

The instructions for your particular test may vary from these. Carefully follow the manual that's included with your device, along with any instructions supplied by your doctor. Be sure to wear the testing unit through the entire night, even if you get up and out of bed, such as to use the bathroom.

Do you have a sleep disorder?

approved a disposable version that includes three small components: a unit you wear on your wrist like a smartwatch and two sensors, one applied to your body and one that slips over your finger. The results of home tests should be interpreted by a sleep medicine specialist.

Actigraphy
Small devices similar to a watch that you wear on your wrist can monitor your motion throughout the day and night. They're programmed with algorithms to differentiate between when you're awake and when you're asleep. Called actigraphy, a test using these devices can help your doctor diagnose disorders involving your circadian rhythm, such as shift work disorder. The test also may be used to help identify sleep patterns in people with insomnia, or to help evaluate hypersomnias. Additionally, the devices can help your doctor assess your treatment and manage your care.

Unlike some other tests, which collect data for just a night or two, actigraphy can provide your physician a longer view of your sleep/wake patterns. You may be asked to wear the device for a few days, or even a couple of weeks.

The devices typically used by physicians have been approved by the FDA after an evaluation of their accuracy. Similar devices that can be purchased over the counter are now used by millions of people. However, they haven't undergone regulatory review and shouldn't be used to diagnose a sleep disorder.

SLEEP SPECIALISTS AND SLEEP CENTERS

As more Americans come to grips with their sleep troubles, and as science makes continued advances in identifying the importance of sleep to good health, the number of medical professionals and facilities treating sleep disorders is on the rise.

Sleep specialists
Sleep specialists are doctors who have specific training in the field of sleep medicine and are certified by the American Board of Sleep Medicine. These individuals have undergone an additional year of

training in a sleep medicine fellowship and have passed a certifying examination. As with other specialties, sleep medicine specialists must refresh their board certification by a maintenance-of-certification process.

Sleep medicine is sometimes referred to as a subspecialty because its physicians are certified in other specialties as well. Sleep specialists come from several different disciplines. Those who treat insomnia and other sleep disorders may be psychiatrists or neurologists. Specialists who treat conditions of the respiratory system, including obstructive sleep apnea, may be pulmonologists or ear, nose and throat specialists (otolaryngologists, or ENTs). Some anesthesiologists also work as sleep specialists, as do some internal or family medicine physicians. And some pediatricians are trained to treat children with sleep disorders.

Sleep centers
Greater interest in sleep medicine has led to the establishment of sleep centers across the country, where interdisciplinary teams of medical professionals work together to diagnose sleep problems.

In addition to a sleep medicine specialist, staff at sleep centers may include nurse practitioners, physician assistants, nurses, sleep technologists and respiratory therapists.

The American Academy of Sleep Medicine is the most common accreditor of sleep centers. To be accredited, a center must be led by a board-certified sleep specialist and meet the academy's standards of care. The academy has an easy-to-use online search tool to locate a sleep center near you (*sleepeducation.org/sleep-center*). There are two main types of sleep centers:
- **Sleep facility.** It includes a clinic for seeing and treating patients and a sleep lab to perform diagnostic tests, such as overnight sleep studies. A sleep facility can also conduct home sleep apnea tests.
- **Independent sleep practice.** This is a sleep clinic that sees and treats patients and conducts home sleep apnea tests. It doesn't have a sleep lab to conduct overnight sleep studies.

When seeking sleep care, look for an accredited sleep center. Your primary care doctor also may refer you to an accredited sleep center for further evaluation, testing or treatment.

6

Insomnia

Michelle had always been a light sleeper. Her sleep became especially poor when she was going through a stressful period, and pregnancy made it difficult to sleep, too. These bouts didn't last long, however, and her sleep would usually improve, seemingly on its own. If she woke in the night, getting a drink of water was usually all it took to help her slip back into sleep.

When she reached her mid-40s and perimenopause, her sleep problems became more persistent. She was feeling stress from a new job, one that included having to make difficult decisions that affected other people. When she lay down in bed, her mind flooded with thoughts of what tomorrow would bring. After eventually falling asleep, she often woke in the night and the thoughts would rush back, again denying her sleep.

Michelle began dreading going to bed. While she lay there, new worries joined her work-related stress, but these new worries were focused on whether she would be able to fall asleep. When she woke in the night, she looked at the clock and became frustrated and anxious about how little time remained before she had to get up. Anxiety about sleep was keeping her from getting what she so desperately desired, in a frustrating, self-fulfilling cycle.

Michelle's sleep deprivation began to affect her daytime functioning. When she woke in the morning without feeling rested, she felt her whole day was shot. She grew irritable. Her depression, which she had long managed, reemerged. She found herself more frequently having a glass or two of wine in the evening, believing it would help her doze off. She soon realized the wine at night was only making her feel worse the next day. After a few months of this, she went to see a doctor and was eventually diagnosed with chronic insomnia.

Michelle's situation is in many ways typical. Insomnia often takes root at stressful moments in life and is nurtured by our own thoughts and actions. Frequently, the way the mind reacts to sleeplessness only makes matters worse. The good news is there are treatments for chronic insomnia that have proven highly successful, whether the problem appears alone or in concert with another mental or physical disorder, as is often the case.

In this chapter, we take an in-depth look at the factors that can contribute to the development of insomnia and the toll the condition can take if ignored. We also review various therapies to treat insomnia that can restore the mental and physical benefits of healthy sleep. Even if your condition seems desperate, there's plenty of reason for hope.

SLEEPLESS IN SEATTLE ... AND ALL OVER

Your body has several ways of letting you know when it's not getting the sleep it needs to perform well and stay healthy. You've likely experienced some of them: A pressing urge to sleep. Waning energy levels and fatigue. Moodiness and irritability. Concentration gaps.

But even when your body is sending clear signals that it's tired and needs rest, you may still struggle to sleep once you turn off the bedroom light.

Insomnia is frustrating and common. Estimates of how many people have insomnia vary. Some reports put it at 1 in 7 U.S. adults. Others suggest it may be as high as 25% of the adult population. What's clear, though, is if you're struggling to sleep, you have plenty of company.

The word *insomnia* comes from the Latin *insomnis,* which means "sleepless." It's the term people typically use to describe difficulty sleeping: nights when you can't fall asleep, when you wake up more times than you can count, or when your eyes fly open well before your alarm clock goes off — and perhaps all three.

It's a safe bet that most of us have experienced occasional insomnia. Bouts of insomnia often occur because of some type of stress in our lives — financial difficulties, concerns at work, a troubled relationship or a health concern. Difficulty sleeping can even result from a *positive* event in life that's also stressful, such as a new job.

> **ARE YOUR MEDICATIONS KEEPING YOU AWAKE?**
>
> Some people find the reason they can't sleep has to do with the pills they're putting in their mouth each day. Many prescription and over-the-counter medications can interfere with sleep and contribute to insomnia.
>
> If your sleep difficulties seem to have emerged about the same time that you added or changed a medication, that may be an important clue. Talk to the doctor who prescribed the drug to see if there may be a link. But don't stop taking the medication without your doctor's approval.
>
> If your sleep troubles align with use of a nonprescription product, such as a supplement or an over-the-counter decongestant, you might want to stop its use and see if your sleep improves. If you're worried about side effects from not taking the product, talk to your doctor first.
>
> For more information on medications that can interfere with sleep, see page 303.

Stress, however, isn't the only culprit. Insomnia may occur for many other reasons — what and when you eat, too little exercise, too much time spent "plugged in," and the list goes on (see Chapter 3).

For many individuals, sleep problems often emerge sometime in their 40s or later, and women are much more likely than men to report trouble sleeping.

Acute vs. chronic insomnia
Not all insomnia is the same. Difficulty sleeping can happen for a short period of time (what's called acute insomnia) or it can persist (what's known as chronic insomnia).

Acute insomnia refers to insomnia symptoms that generally occur less than three times a week, or insomnia that's been a problem for less than three months. In many instances of acute insomnia, fitful nights in bed gradually fade over a period of two or three months. Perhaps the stressful situation resolves itself, or you become more resilient and the problem seems less concerning.

This is different from insomnia that becomes more prevalent with time or that lingers. When insomnia symptoms don't resolve after a few months, they probably won't disappear on their own anytime soon. Insomnia that occurs at least three times a week and lasts more than three months is considered chronic insomnia.

The transition from acute to chronic insomnia is the result of a complex interplay of factors and involves more than just the passing of time. Chronic insomnia can happen for several reasons, including illness, medications, poor sleep habits, stress, and anxiety about not being able to sleep. Concerns related to lack of sleep and its consequences can become obsessive, only perpetuating the problem.

The medical term for insomnia is insomnia disorder. While many people have difficulty sleeping, a much smaller number are diagnosed with insomnia disorder. To receive a diagnosis of insomnia disorder, you must display the following: difficulty falling asleep, staying asleep or sustaining quality sleep, as well as feeling fatigued or sleepy during the day and experiencing impairment or distress at work or at home.

Each year, 6% to 10% of U.S. adults receive a diagnosis of insomnia disorder. The table on the next page outlines signs and symptoms and other qualifiers that doctors look for to make an insomnia diagnosis.

INTERNATIONAL CLASSIFICATION OF SLEEP DISORDERS, THIRD EDITION (ICSD-3) DIAGNOSTIC CRITERIA FOR CHRONIC INSOMNIA DISORDER

Diagnostic criteria A-F must be met:

A	The patient reports, or the patient's parent or caregiver observes, one or more of the following: • Difficulty initiating sleep[a] • Difficulty maintaining sleep[b] • Waking up earlier than desired[c] • Resistance to going to bed on appropriate schedule • Difficulty sleeping without parent or caregiver intervention
B	The patient reports, or the patient's parent or caregiver observes, one or more of the following related to the nighttime sleep difficulty: • Fatigue/malaise • Attention, concentration or memory impairment • Impaired social, family, occupational or academic performance • Mood disturbance/irritability • Daytime sleepiness • Behavioral problems (e.g., hyperactivity, impulsivity, aggression) • Reduced motivation/energy/initiative • Proneness to errors/accidents • Concerns about or dissatisfaction with sleep
C	The reported sleep-wake complaints cannot be explained purely by inadequate opportunity (i.e., enough time is allotted for sleep) or inadequate circumstances (i.e., the environment is safe, dark, quiet and comfortable) for sleep
D	The sleep disturbance and associated daytime symptoms occur at least three times per week
E	The sleep disturbance and associated daytime symptoms have been present for at least three months
F	The sleep-wake difficulty is not better explained by another sleep disorder

[a]In general, delays of >20 minutes for children and young adults and >30 minutes for middle-aged and older adults are considered clinically significant.

[b]In general, periods of awakening in the middle of the night of >20 minutes for children and young adults and >30 minutes for middle-aged and older adults are considered clinically significant.

[c]In general, waking up >30 minutes before normal awakening time is considered clinically significant.

Reproduced with permission.

THE HUGE TOLL OF INSOMNIA

Insomnia is more than a nighttime problem — it affects you at all hours of the day. It can diminish your quality of life, decrease your vitality and cloud your mental performance. Individuals with insomnia tend to be absent from work more often and their productivity at work decreases. Data also indicates that if you have insomnia, you're 2.5 to 4.5 times more likely to have an accident.

Then there's the effect on your health. Insomnia places you at greater risk of several health problems. Sleep loss is associated with diseases and conditions such as obesity, diabetes, high blood pressure, increased infections, reduced cognitive functioning and even death (see Chapter 3).

Beyond your individual well-being, insomnia can have a profound effect on your family and your relationships. Individuals who are sleep-deprived are more likely to react poorly in social situations and to experience increased feelings of loneliness, isolation or depression. Relationships with family often become strained.

The societal costs associated with insomnia are estimated in the billions of dollars largely due to greater demands on healthcare, lost productivity and an increase in accidents.

WHY INSOMNIA DEVELOPS

Sleep might have come easily to you for many years, then changed, gradually or suddenly, into a maddening problem. Exactly why this happens varies from person to person, and the underlying causes can be difficult to pin down.

Experts have found some commonalities, however, and they tend to approach insomnia as a combination of ingredients coming together at a specific time to disrupt sleep.

These ingredients often include underlying risk factors for insomnia combined with stressful or disruptive life circumstances or events. The result is a change in sleep, along with worries about being able to sleep. The combination can lead to unhealthy habits, exacerbating the problem.

The three Ps

Sleep experts sometimes refer to the risk for developing insomnia in terms of "three Ps." The three Ps model suggests that certain predisposing, precipitating and perpetuating factors contribute to the sleep disorder. This framework takes into account that how you respond to periods of sleeplessness might actually contribute to the problem.

Predisposing

Some people are simply more likely to develop insomnia than others. Women are typically at greater risk than men. Family history also can play a role, with some people being genetically predisposed to the condition. Daily circumstances, including working the night shift or sleeping with a bed partner who snores or tosses and turns, can make you more prone to poor sleep. Predisposing factors don't cause insomnia but can set the stage.

INSOMNIA AND DEPRESSION

Does insomnia cause depression? Or the reverse: Does depression lead to insomnia?

Approximately 40% of people with insomnia also have a mental health disorder, most commonly depression. In some people, depression comes first and trouble sleeping follows. In others, insomnia is eventually accompanied by depression.

Despite appearances, it's not always clear whether the first condition to emerge causes the other.

There's good evidence suggesting that depression and insomnia can share underlying causes, with each developing independently, though simultaneously. For example, problems with regulation of the body's stress hormone cortisol can contribute to either depression or insomnia.

Successful treatment generally involves addressing both conditions.

Precipitating

For people who are predisposed to insomnia, even something small can trigger sleep troubles. If you tend to have trouble sleeping, the story about a princess who couldn't sleep because of a tiny pea beneath her mattresses might not sound like a fairy tale at all.

Among individuals who aren't predisposed to poor sleep, traumatic events such as the death of a loved one, a divorce or the loss of a job can bring on sleep problems. In some cases, these precipitating factors can be cumulative, with multiple stresses building up and pushing you toward insomnia.

Perpetuating

When sleeplessness does occur because of predisposing and precipitating factors, it often resolves itself, perhaps over several weeks or a couple of months. Sometimes, though, how you respond to sleep troubles may perpetuate the problem. You may begin to take naps during the day, drink more coffee to stay alert or alcohol to help you sleep. Or you may spend nights you can't sleep surfing the web on your cell phone or computer.

Choices such as these can make it more difficult to fall asleep, prompting you to grow increasingly anxious as you lie awake. You may begin to spend more time in bed, thinking this will surely help you get the sleep you need. But the additional time in bed only adds to the angst, and your body begins to associate your bed with anxiety, not rest. These reactions are completely understandable, but they can lead to long-term problems sleeping.

The sleep-wake balance

In addition to the "three Ps," sleep experts have developed other ways of thinking about insomnia, creating models to help guide research and treatment. One such model is known as circadian and homeostatic sleep regulation. Here's how it works.

In a sense, being awake makes you sleepy. This is because the longer you're awake, the more tired you become. During the day, you're constantly adding to this pressure to sleep, which becomes one of the primary forces urging you to turn in for the night. This process is referred to as sleep homeostasis.

At the same time, humans and other living creatures experience physiological cycles during the day known as circadian rhythms. These cycles, or rhythms, are an evolutionary adaptation to the fact that we live on a planet that has night and day. There are advantages to being awake and active during daylight, and to resting at night so that your body and brain can conduct routine maintenance — the basic role of sleep. Your circadian rhythms drive you toward sleep at night and keep you alert during the day.

During a 24-hour day, your homeostatic and circadian systems work in sync, regulating the processes that keep you awake, as well as those that orchestrate sleep. These systems are kept in exquisite balance: As processes slow on one side of the sleep-wake scale, others engage on the opposite side. During daytime, your body is kept awake and alert. With night approaching, the processes that keep you active begin to wind down, and you get sleepy.

Under healthy conditions, this choreographed balance between sleep and wakefulness goes unnoticed. Sometimes, though, the balance is disrupted. When this happens, the systems stop working in harmony and begin to produce friction and conflict. Pressure to sleep naturally rises during the day to make you sleepy, but the systems that keep you awake fail to disengage as they should.

You find yourself both sleepy and alert — "tired but wired," as it's sometimes described. The result is a poor night's sleep that leaves you unrestored and less resilient the next day.

WHEN TO SEE A DOCTOR

Fortunately, insomnia is often short-lived, and healthy sleep returns. For a while, your difficulties sleeping may seem stubbornly persistent, but they eventually dissipate and resolve within a month or two. Sometimes the improvement happens on its own. Other times, it's in response to lifestyle changes and improved sleep habits, actions you take to help you sleep better.

In some instances, though, insomnia symptoms don't fade and are still present after more than three months, with a significant impact on your life. At this point, the sleeplessness likely won't go away anytime soon, and you should look at it as an ongoing problem that needs to be addressed.

Unfortunately, many people don't seek medical care, and their insomnia goes undiagnosed and untreated. By some estimates, only one-quarter to one-half of people with symptoms of insomnia discuss them with their doctors. Insomnia is generally a treatable condition, but medical treatment can't begin without seeing a healthcare professional.

If you're experiencing ongoing sleep problems that you've been unable to resolve and the problems are affecting your daily life, it's time

---

CONSIDER THE ODDS

As you might expect, many people struggling to sleep often turn to the internet to see if they can figure out what's wrong with them. And some come across a condition called fatal insomnia. Without the proper context, this can be an alarming experience.

Known medically as fatal familial insomnia, this inherited disorder is caused by a specific genetic mutation that's very uncommon. It's so rare, in fact, that fewer than 40 cases per year are reported. For comparison, by some estimates up to 70 million Americans have ongoing sleep difficulties that occur for other reasons.

Early symptoms of fatal insomnia can include a decrease in the time spent sleeping and increasingly vivid dreams. As it progresses, the condition can cause weight loss, a change in gait, double vision, mood changes and delirium, eventually leading to death.

Don't let yourself assume that because you can't sleep you have fatal insomnia. The odds are overwhelming that you don't. However, if you do experience symptoms such as weight loss, a change in gait or double vision, make sure to see a doctor. They all warrant medical attention.

to make that appointment. You can begin by visiting with your family doctor or by seeing a sleep specialist, if one is available.

DIAGNOSING INSOMNIA

There's no blood test that can signal that you have insomnia and no imaging technology that can reveal it. Instead, a diagnosis of insomnia disorder comes primarily from conversations between you, your doctor and your medical team. Diagnosing insomnia disorder generally involves a detailed exploration of your symptoms and ruling out other conditions that could be causing them.

EARLY STEPS TO BETTER SLEEP

There are several changes that you can make on your own now to help you start sleeping better (see Chapter 4). A good place to begin is with these proven healthy sleep habits:

- **Stick to a regular sleep schedule.** Keep your bedtime and wake time consistent from day to day, including on weekends.
- **Minimize stimulation before bedtime.** This includes turning off devices and screens and developing a routine that allows you time to wind down.
- **Make your bedroom an inviting place to sleep.** Keep it dark, cool and quiet.
- **Develop skills to help you relax more and stress less.** Proven relaxation techniques that help promote sleep include mindfulness practices such as meditation and guided imagery.
- **Cut back on substances that interfere with sleep.** Avoid alcohol and caffeine several hours before bed. It's best to eliminate nicotine altogether.

To gain a complete picture of your sleep troubles, you'll likely be asked a variety of questions about your symptoms and to fill out one or more questionnaires pertaining to various aspects of your sleep. For more information on questionnaires used to help evaluate insomnia, see pages 115 and 117.

Questionnaire topics or conversations with team members may include:
- Your health history, including current diseases and conditions.
- Medications you take.
- Your use of caffeine, alcohol and other substances.
- How you prepare for bed, how long it takes you to fall asleep and how often you wake in the night.
- Your level of daytime fatigue and sleepiness.
- How poor sleep affects your daily life.

You also may be asked to complete a two-week sleep diary, including what time you went to bed, when you fell asleep, how often you woke up during the night, when you woke for the last time and what time you got out of bed. Sleep diaries may also be used after a diagnosis of insomnia disorder to help track improvement in your sleep.

In addition to determining if you have insomnia and its potential root causes, information gained in the diagnostic process can help identify if the insomnia is appearing on its own or in tandem with another condition.

It's not uncommon for insomnia disorder to be diagnosed with another condition. For instance, insomnia and obstructive sleep apnea are sometimes diagnosed together. According to one study, 1 in 10 individuals with insomnia also has obstructive sleep apnea, and 4 in 10 people with sleep apnea were also diagnosed as having insomnia. Together, the conditions are sometimes called comorbid insomnia and sleep apnea (COMISA).

Additional tests

Depending on your situation, a diagnosis of insomnia disorder and the search for its cause may require that you undergo certain tests or exams. These may include:

Physical exam
If the cause of your insomnia is unknown, your doctor may perform a physical exam to look for signs of medical problems that may be related to your condition.

Sleep study
If you have signs of another sleep disorder, such as sleep apnea or unusual movement during sleep, you may be asked to undergo a sleep study (polysomnography). A sleep study monitors and records a variety of body activities while you sleep, including brain waves, breathing, heartbeat, eye movements and body movements. See the illustration on page 119.

The American Academy of Sleep Medicine doesn't recommend a sleep study in the routine evaluation of insomnia. However, if you snore or have been told you sometimes make snorting sounds during the night, that could be a sign of a breathing problem, and a sleep study may be used to rule out other causes.

Actigraphy
This test may be requested if your doctor wants to learn more about your sleep and wake patterns to help determine if an issue with your circadian rhythms could be affecting your sleep. With this test, you wear a device that measures your movements. Actigraphy is also sometimes used when diagnosing insomnia related to depression.

FINDING HOPE IN TREATMENT

In the darkness of night, insomnia may seem unbeatable, but, in fact, the condition is often treatable, and improvements can be long-lasting. People who see a doctor and take steps to address their sleep problems often reduce or eliminate their symptoms altogether and can begin enjoying the many benefits of improved sleep.

Changing sleep habits and addressing issues that may be associated with insomnia, such as stress or poor sleep habits, can restore restful sleep for many people. If these measures alone aren't enough, your doctor may recommend cognitive behavioral therapy, medication or a combination of therapy and medication to improve your sleep.

Cognitive behavioral therapy for insomnia (CBT-I) is considered the first-line treatment because of its high success rate and lasting results. This is a multipronged therapy with the goal of refocusing your thinking and behaviors regarding sleep.

In cases where CBT-I isn't producing the desired result, a medication that helps promote sleep may be introduced into treatment. Medication also may be prescribed when short-term benefits are needed, such as during a time of grief or extraordinary stress. How best to use sleep medications, their risks and benefits, and when they may be combined with CBT-I are discussed in detail in the next chapter.

When you begin treatment for insomnia, don't be afraid to ask questions, especially if you don't feel comfortable with the treatment plan presented to you. If you have long-term insomnia symptoms and your doctor recommends only medication, inquire about other treatments, including CBT-I. Question your doctor further if your treatment plan only addresses improving your sleep habits (sleep hygiene). Such a limited approach to treatment isn't considered adequate for chronic insomnia. The American Academy of Sleep Medicine emphasizes this point, stating that CBT-I or some other type of behavioral component is recommended in the treatment of insomnia disorder.

COGNITIVE BEHAVIORAL THERAPY FOR INSOMNIA (CBT-I)

The most effective, lasting treatment for insomnia is cognitive behavioral therapy for insomnia. The treatment has been in use for decades and is time proven. The purpose of CBT-I treatment is to improve sleep by changing the way people think and act regarding sleep. CBT-I may be administered by several different trained, certified healthcare professionals, including therapists, psychologists, sleep physicians or nurses.

Data indicates that CBT-I is effective in 70% to 80% of those who try it, and the results tend to be long-lasting, without the need for additional treatment. CBT-I treatment is generally preferred to use of sleeping pills because of its durability, and it's more successful when performed alone than in conjunction with medication. In fact, reducing the need for sleep medication is considered one of the advantages of CBT-I.

How it works
To understand CBT-I, it's best to think of it not as a single therapy; rather, picture it as a suite of treatments — specific actions and educational components brought together to improve your sleep. Treatment may vary somewhat from therapist to therapist and clinic to clinic, but it generally focuses on changing behaviors and thought patterns that are conspiring to keep you awake when you should be sleeping. While it may sound like a yearslong process, it's not. Successful treatment often can be accomplished in 6 to 8 sessions.

In the remainder of this chapter, we discuss in detail specific therapies involved in CBT-I. Core components of the approach include stimulus control therapy, sleep restriction therapy, cognitive therapy, sleep hygiene and relaxation therapies. Some of these practices involve learning new skills, which often takes practice, both during therapy sessions and at home. A few of the steps might leave you feeling drowsy and fatigued during the day. This usually gets better quickly.

Keep in mind that the improvements in sleep from CBT-I can be gradual and they may take time to become apparent. You should have realistic expectations when you begin the therapy and not lose patience if a few weeks pass with what appear to be small gains. It's important to stick with the treatment, as this relatively modest investment of time and effort holds the promise of lasting benefits.

There are self-guided and online versions of CBT-I treatment available; however, most studies have demonstrated that in-person CBT-I is best. That said, if group treatment or online programs are the only option or the best available option in your circumstances, don't rule them out. Talk with your doctor about the best route for you.

Stimulus control therapy
One of the most famous experiments in psychology involved dogs, a bell and a Russian scientist named Ivan Petrovich Pavlov. Pavlov rang the bell every time the dogs were fed. At first they had no reaction.

After a while, though, the sound of the bell prompted the dogs to salivate. The dogs didn't decide to do this; their bodies responded involuntarily in anticipation of being fed. Pavlov demonstrated that the body can react to a stimulus with an involuntary physical response, what's called classical conditioning.

Stimulus control therapy is based on classical conditioning, and it's a core concept of CBT-I. Just as a dog comes to associate the sound of a bell with food so strongly that it salivates, the goal is to make the association between your bed and sleep so strong that you become sleepy when you lie down. To reinforce this association, it's important you only use your bed for sleeping or sex. The more you use it for other

STIMULUS CONTROL THERAPY TO-DO LIST

If you want to try stimulus control, take these steps:
- Go to bed when you're sleepy and get up at the same time every morning.
- Get out of bed after 10 minutes if you can't fall asleep or if you wake up and can't get back to sleep.
- Sit upright in a chair or couch and do something that relaxes you. Read a nonstimulating book or magazine, do a crossword or sudoku puzzle, play solitaire, knit or listen to a guided meditation.
- Once your eyes are heavy and you feel sleepy, hang in there a while longer until your urge to sleep is strong. Then return to bed.

Things to avoid:
- Reading or watching television in bed.
- Interacting with screens when you get out of bed because you can't sleep.
- Taking naps during the day.
- Sleeping longer than eight hours.

things — doing work on your laptop, watching TV, visiting on your phone — the weaker that association becomes.

Stimulus control therapy includes a few simple rules: Go to bed only when you're sleepy. If you haven't fallen asleep within about 10 minutes, get out of bed and do something relaxing, such as reading in low light or listening to a guided meditation. Some people simply sit in a comfortable chair and stare off at nothing. Don't look at your phone or computer or TV. Once you begin to feel sleepy, wait just a bit longer, then return to bed.

Follow the same routine if you wake in the middle of the night and can't fall asleep within about 10 minutes. An important note: Don't look at a clock. Instead guess when you think about 10 minutes have elapsed. Staring at a clock to time how long it takes to fall asleep doesn't help the situation.

Stimulus control also involves a couple of other key actions: establishing a consistent time for waking up in the morning and avoiding naps.

These actions take just a bit of effort. Don't be discouraged if you feel tired and drowsy when sitting down but find yourself unable to sleep in bed. Your body will learn. Also, you may feel sleep-deprived during the day. Stick with it, though, and this will be an important step toward improving your sleep.

Sleep restriction therapy
A common reaction to sleeping poorly is to spend more time in bed. The longer you're in bed, the greater the opportunity to sleep, right? Surprisingly, this can have the opposite effect and instead make it more difficult to fall asleep.

The important principle here is that the sleepier you are, the better your chances of falling asleep. Sleep restriction therapy works to build up that pressure to sleep — your homeostatic sleep drive — to help you doze off faster. The American Academy of Sleep Medicine recommends using sleep restriction as one element of CBT-I. In some cases, however, sleep restriction therapy may be used alone.

To begin the therapy, your doctor will give you what might be called a sleep prescription. It's not a pill but a recommended length of time for you to spend in bed each night.

Here's an example of how sleep restriction works: Prior to treatment, you were going to bed at 9 p.m. each night, taking two hours to fall asleep, waking at 5 a.m., and then finally getting out of bed at 6 a.m. to get ready for work. Out of the nine hours you were in bed, only six were spent sleeping. Your sleep efficiency — or the ratio of hours asleep to hours in bed, expressed as a percentage — was 66%, which is low.

To remedy this, your doctor gives you a sleep prescription of six hours: Go to bed at midnight and get out of bed at 6 a.m., regardless of how much of that time you spend sleeping. The next day, you might feel slightly sleep-deprived, and in this case that's good. This sleep pressure helps make you sleepy at bedtime. Think of it like hunger: Just as dinner tastes better if you sit down at the table when you're hungry, sleep comes more easily if you get into bed when you're sleepy.

When the time you're asleep closely matches the time spent in bed, your sleep prescription is gradually increased, perhaps in 15-minute increments. Your goal is to have a sleep efficiency of at least 85%. As an

SLEEP RESTRICTION THERAPY TO-DO LIST

If you want to try this, take these steps:
- Limit your time in bed to the average amount you're currently sleeping. (Don't limit your time to less than five hours.)
- Set your sleep window — the time you can sleep — based on your desired wake time, then determine your bedtime.
- Don't go to bed before your set bedtime.
- Go to bed only when you're sleepy or your sleep urge is highest.
- If you have trouble settling your mind and falling asleep, get out of bed and do something relaxing until you're really ready to sleep.
- Get up at the same time every day.
- Don't nap.

example, spending eight hours in bed and sleeping for seven hours is slightly above that goal.

There are other important elements of sleep restriction therapy. One is avoiding naps, which reduce nighttime sleepiness. Another is establishing consistent bedtimes and wake times, which helps stabilize your body's circadian rhythms.

If you share a bed with a partner, you might ask that person to sleep elsewhere during this crucial part of this treatment. Doing so may reduce interruptions for both of you and help the process along. In the end, both partners benefit when each is sleeping well.

Because sleep restriction therapy relies in part on daytime drowsiness to bring on sleep at night, it may not be appropriate for some people, including drivers or heavy machinery operators. It also may not be suited for people with some mental health conditions, such as mania, hypomania or seizure disorders.

Cognitive therapy

Sleep is one of those things that only get more difficult the harder you try. Lying in bed and obsessing about how you can't sleep is one of the surest ways to fail in your sleep attempts.

Cognitive therapy is the component of CBT-I that focuses on your thinking. Its purpose is to teach you to recognize negative thoughts and worries, and then take steps to restructure them.

As you lie sleepless in bed, your mind can conjure up a swarm of negative, inaccurate thoughts and the possibility of dire outcomes, what psychologists call catastrophizing: *I'll never get to sleep! It's getting later and later, and my time to sleep is getting shorter and shorter! My day will be ruined! I'll be lousy at work, and I'll lose my job! I need a sleeping pill!*

Cognitive therapy teaches you to recognize that these are inaccurate, counterproductive thoughts, and it trains you to replace them with reasoning that's accurate and positive: *I will get to sleep. My day tomorrow won't be ruined. My job is not on the line. I can fall asleep without a sleeping pill.*

With practice and time, cognitive restructuring becomes ingrained and your thinking more positive and less of a hindrance to sleep.

COGNITIVE BEHAVIORAL THERAPY AND ITS BEGINNINGS

Cognitive behavioral therapy for insomnia is one of many branches of cognitive behavioral therapy (CBT), a widely accepted approach to address several psychological conditions. Cognitive behavioral therapy emerged in the 1960s and '70s as psychiatrists and psychologists began combining two separate threads of research and treatment in their field, cognitive therapy and behavioral therapy.

American psychiatrist Aaron Beck played a crucial role in bringing these schools of thought together and is widely considered to be the founder of cognitive behavioral therapy. Importantly, he focused the therapy on addressing individual problems, not on a person's overall psychological state or history, as is the practice with some types of long-term psychotherapy.

Beck's early efforts were focused on treating depression, the most common condition among his patients at the time. From the outset, he validated the results with randomized controlled trials, the gold standard in scientific research. There are now hundreds of such studies supporting the effectiveness of CBT for depression, anxiety, substance abuse, marital problems, eating disorders and other disorders, including insomnia. CBT has become one of the most widely used and accepted approaches to psychological care.

The treatment is based on a few core concepts. One is that flawed or negative thinking contributes to psychological problems. Another is that these problems are also exacerbated by our learned unhelpful behaviors. By changing both thinking and behavior, people can learn to better deal with or even overcome their psychological problems.

CBT is sometimes referred to as action-oriented or problem-focused treatment. In addition to recognizing negative or irrational thoughts, it offers coping skills to change thinking and behavior.

Sleep hygiene
Sleep hygiene is a term often used to describe efforts to improve sleep by addressing habits, behaviors and environmental factors that can interfere with sleep. Some sleep problems may be associated with years of unhealthy sleep routines.

To help improve your ability to fall asleep and stay asleep, you need to look at specific things you do — or don't do — that may be contributing to the problem. Unhealthy sleep habits and how to address them are discussed in Chapter 4.

Relaxation therapies
There are several things you can do to relax and reduce some of the mental stimulation that may be keeping you awake. Relaxation therapies are often helpful in promoting sleep and are another component of CBT-I.

Practices that may be used in the treatment of insomnia include meditation, guided imagery, relaxed breathing and progressive muscle relaxation.

Meditation
Meditation refers to a group of techniques with a common goal of helping you to focus your attention on the present moment. This may be done by repeating a word or a phrase, with specific body movements or by focusing intently on your breathing. Mindfulness is a type of meditation in which you focus on your immediate surroundings, sensations and feelings, without judgment.

The idea behind meditation is to interrupt the stream of thoughts that normally occupies the conscious mind. Doing so can lead to a state of relaxation, mental calmness and psychological balance.

Practicing meditation may help you control how you respond to a challenging situation, in this case insomnia. Studies validate that meditation can help reduce insomnia symptoms.

Guided imagery
This mindfulness technique uses the power of imagination to help your body relax. You visualize a peaceful setting with your mind's eye and use all your senses to imagine yourself there. Your brain receives

messages from this imagined setting that help your body relax, just as if you were actually there.

Similar to other forms of relaxation therapy, guided imagery may help to reduce your stress level and calm your mind before bed.

Relaxed breathing
Relaxed, or deep, breathing is a technique that helps you breathe more efficiently. It involves deep, even-paced breathing using your diaphragm

---

A SIMPLE MEDITATION EXERCISE

If you want to try meditation, take these steps:
- **Make yourself comfortable.** You want to feel relaxed but alert.
- **Soften your gaze.** You can close your eyes or rest them lightly on something a few feet in front of you.
- **Become aware that you are sitting.** Feel the sensations of your body being supported. Remind yourself that you do not have to be anywhere else at this time.
- **Now bring your attention to your breath.** Focus on the rhythm of your breath as air moves in and out of your body. Notice the rise and fall of your chest and belly. Become aware of any tensions you are holding in your body and let them relax with each breath.
- **Your mind may wander from time to time.** Gently draw your attention back to your breath. Each time this happens, begin again without judgment.
- **At first you may meditate for as little as a few minutes a couple of times a day.** As you end your meditation, briefly thank yourself for taking this time to focus on you.
- **You may also choose to add a mantra.** This can be a prayer or a word that you focus on with each breath. Examples are words such as *calm, peace, strength* and *joy*.

to expand your lungs and take in more oxygen. Breathing in this manner is also relaxing and is a helpful technique for relieving tension and stress. Most people don't breathe deeply, especially when they're stressed.

Learning how to take deep, slow breaths can help lessen your stress level, helping you to sleep better. Deep breathing can be practiced most anywhere.

A GUIDED IMAGERY EXERCISE

If you want to try guided imagery, take these steps:

- **Relax.** Clear your mind of all chatter, worries and distractions by filling your thoughts with kindness and love. Loosen any tight-fitting clothing and find a comfortable, quiet place. Begin taking slow, deep breaths through your nose down into your belly. Imagine you're breathing in self-kindness and breathing out some of your tension.
- **Concentrate.** Focus your attention on your slow, deep breathing as you clear your mind. Try placing one hand on your belly and feel it rise with each deep breath in and then fall with each breath out. If your mind wanders, acknowledge the thoughts that enter your mind and send yourself kindness and compassion.
- **Visualize.** For the next several minutes, visualize yourself healthy, happy and whole and in a relaxing setting. You might imagine yourself at the beach, enjoying a walk in the woods or simply spending quiet time in your favorite chair.
- **Affirm.** Choose an affirmation or words that are sacred for you as you continue to see yourself as healthy, happy and whole. This positive affirmation and image of you will help plant the seeds for your healing. Whenever you feel challenged, remember this image and affirmation to take you back to a state of calm relaxation.

Progressive muscle relaxation

Progressive muscle relaxation is designed to reduce stress and anxiety by reducing tension in your muscles. The technique focuses on slow, steady shortening (tensing) of a muscle, followed by a gradual relaxation phase in which you lengthen and relax the muscle. You might begin with the muscles in your toes and feet and work your way up to those in your head and face.

A RELAXED BREATHING EXERCISE

If you want to try relaxed breathing, take these steps:
- Find a quiet place where you can sit or lie comfortably.
- Stretch out your shoulders and arms, then let your shoulders relax and drop.
- Breathe in slowly through your nose until you feel comfortably full. This could be to a count of four, for example. Think about breathing from your belly, so it moves out as you breathe in.
- Hold your breath for four seconds or so, then slowly exhale. Breathe out slowly and smoothly to the count of four. Let your belly flatten. When you breathe from your belly you'll be able to keep your chest still and your shoulders relaxed.

Tips for best results:
- Slow, smooth, even breathing is best. If you wish, place one hand on your upper chest and the other hand on your belly. This helps you feel your muscles as you breathe.
- Think of your belly like a balloon. It gets bigger as you inhale and smaller as you exhale.
- Repeat this skill as often as needed. At first it may feel awkward. But keep practicing until it feels natural and relaxing. You can use this skill alone or with other relaxation methods.

A PROGRESSIVE MUSCLE RELAXATION EXERCISE

If you want to try muscle relaxation, take these steps:
- Find a quiet place where you can lie or sit down. Loosen any tight clothing and get comfortable.
- Work on only one group of muscles at a time (see below). Keep the rest of your body relaxed.
- Tighten all the muscles in that group.
- Hold the muscles tight for 5 seconds or for a count of eight. Notice how it feels as you tighten the muscles.
- Release the tightness in those muscles. Note the difference between the tight state and the relaxed state. Relax for 30 seconds.
- Tighten the same muscle group a second time and then move on to the next muscle group.

Work on each part of your body. You can begin with your feet and toes and work upward. Or you can start with your head and face and move downward.

Here's what to do:
- **Feet and toes.** Curl the toes downward, as if you're trying to tightly grip something with them.
- **Thighs and calves.** Tighten the muscles in your lower legs (calves) and your upper legs (thighs).
- **Chest, stomach and back.** Do all these areas together. Hold your breath and try to pull your belly button down to your spine.
- **Arms and hands.** Make fists and tighten every muscle in your arms.
- **Neck and shoulders.** Lift your shoulders toward your ears and tighten your neck as you do it.
- **Head and face.** Clench your jaw. Scrunch your eyes and your forehead.

This relaxation skill teaches you what tight muscles feel like — and what it feels like when you're totally relaxed. Knowing that difference can help you find stress spots in your body so that you can release the tension before you go to bed.

Additional tools and techniques
Sometimes additional therapies are included as part of CBT-I or the length of treatment is altered.

Phototherapy
If your insomnia is due in part to a disruption in your body's natural circadian rhythms, CBT-I may include the use of phototherapy. Phototherapy, sometimes called bright-light therapy, uses bright light to help sync your body's internal clock with day and night. Bright light first thing in the morning can help to establish healthy circadian rhythms.

Phototherapy may require use of a special, full-spectrum light or another means of stimulating your eyes for 30 minutes or more. In some cases, and at certain times of year, natural sunlight may be sufficient.

Phototherapy is generally most effective when it's used in conjunction with other therapies to treat insomnia. As a stand-alone treatment, it's been shown to improve only a few measures of sleep quality, not all of them.

Brief therapies
While CBT-I can efficiently bring improvement in 6 to 8 sessions, there are instances in which a shorter course of treatment might be preferable. Brief therapies for insomnia apply some elements of CBT-I but in just four sessions. This approach may be appropriate for people who find it difficult to complete the full course, and it addresses the shortage of clinicians trained in CBT-I.

A truncated treatment plan still employs training in sleep restriction (limiting the time in bed to the time you sleep) and stimulus control (avoiding the bed for anything but sleep or sex). It typically entails two in-person sessions and two telephone sessions to check on your progress and to make adjustments.

The first session is the most involved and can last an hour or more, while the others may be shorter, perhaps 30 minutes or less. The first session teaches four "rules" derived from sleep restriction therapy:
- Reduce your time in bed.
- Wake up at the same time every day.
- Go to bed only when sleepy.
- Don't stay in bed unless you're asleep.

Studies of middle-aged and older adults show that a shortened treatment plan produces results similar to CBT-I, though some of the improvements are slightly smaller when compared with a standard treatment plan.

CBT-I APPS: AN ALTERNATIVE FOR SOME

Several apps and online courses are now available that deliver an interactive version of CBT-I through your phone, tablet or laptop, and for some people these can be a good option.

Apps use combinations of text, videos, quizzes, exercises and vignettes. They often include many of the usual elements of CBT-I, such as sleep restriction, stimulus control, relaxation training and cognitive therapy.

Studies indicate that users of these apps fell asleep faster, stayed asleep longer and improved their sleep efficiency when compared with individuals who did nothing. One review of the research found the effectiveness of CBT-I apps was similar to in-person visits with a therapist.

However, many users don't stick with the app and stop using it. If you use a CBT-I app, know that there might come a time when you become less engaged, and you'll need to work through that to continue to benefit from the program. Individuals who stuck with an app generally found long-term improvements in their sleep.

Finding CBT-I treatment

You can find medical institutions and individual practitioners who specialize in sleep treatments and are accredited by the American Academy of Sleep Medicine at *sleepeducation.org*. To be accredited, the center's healthcare team must be led by a board-certified physician; however, you might see someone other than a doctor for your treatment, such as a therapist or a nurse.

The Society of Behavioral Sleep Medicine, which promotes treatments based on CBT, has a directory of therapists on its website at *behavioralsleep.org*.

Clinicians trained specifically in CBT-I are in great demand, and in some parts of the country it can be difficult to get an appointment. Often, a therapist who practices CBT but isn't a specialist in sleep medicine can offer a similar treatment. Group sessions also work very well for many people, and wider acceptance of telemedicine has made it easier to find and meet with a therapist.

Some people benefit from self-help methods based on CBT-I treatment. A randomized, controlled trial of people with insomnia who were given a self-help book that included information on CBT-I and how to implement it improved their sleep and reduced their use of sleep medication. Many apps are now available that provide a course of CBT-I.

WHEN MEDICATION MAY BE PART OF TREATMENT

While cognitive behavioral therapy is typically the first-line treatment for insomnia and has a high success rate, medications are sometimes prescribed to help improve sleep. Prescription pills can help you get to sleep, stay asleep or both. Doctors generally don't recommend relying on prescription sleeping pills for more than a few weeks, but several medications are approved for long-term use.

If you're prescribed a sleep medication as part of your treatment, learning how various drugs work will help you better understand the recommendation your doctor is making. Knowing the history of sleep medications is instructive, too, because it helps explain why some sleeping pills have a less-than-positive reputation.

The next chapter offers detailed information on medications used to treat sleep disorders, including insomnia. Like many drugs, sleep medications can be beneficial if taken for the right reasons, in the right amount, and for the right length of time, but they also carry significant risks if not taken properly.

7

Sleep medications

During one of those nights when you're struggling to sleep, taking a sleeping pill might seem like a good solution. Sleep medications have some legitimate uses. They can provide immediate benefits to help you during a particularly difficult period in life, or as a bridge while you try to break a bad sleep pattern and adopt healthier habits.

But it's important not to overlook the fact that many sleep medications carry significant risks. They may provide a temporary fix, but generally aren't a long-term solution. If you're considering taking a sleeping pill or one has been prescribed for you, learn everything about it to avoid potentially serious side effects and misuse of the medication.

PROPER USE OF SLEEP MEDICATIONS

Pharmaceutical researchers have developed several different ways to induce sleep, leading to dozens of sleep medications — with sometimes confusing names. Many of these medications are based upon a few different strategies that work on specific signaling systems in the brain. Each approach has advantages and disadvantages, depending on the person taking the medication and their individual sleep problems.

Some of the most commonly prescribed medications to induce sleep have been around for decades, and some have fallen out of favor because of their undesirable side effects.

If medication becomes part of your treatment for insomnia, work with your doctor to determine the best option for you. The drug prescribed should be selected to match you and your sleep issues, including whether you have trouble falling asleep, staying asleep, waking too early or some combination of these. Other mental or physical conditions that may be contributing to your sleep problems, as well as other medications you're already taking, also need to be taken into consideration.

Medication may be included in insomnia treatment in cases of extreme stress or grief or when current therapies aren't providing enough benefit. When used appropriately, medications can help some people with stubborn insomnia symptoms improve their sleep and their overall health and quality of life.

If medications do become part of your treatment, it may become necessary to adjust the dosage or switch to a related medication to get the results you want. Don't ever change doses on your own, and don't stop taking the medication without first consulting with your doctor. Doing so can cause anxiety and worsen insomnia symptoms.

SLEEP MEDICATIONS EXPLAINED

The human brain is a magnificent signaling machine, using electrical impulses and chemical messages to shuttle information from cell to cell. This is not only how your brain thinks and remembers but also how it sends commands to all the basic operating systems in your body.

One way your brain sends and receives messages is with specialized chemicals, called neurotransmitters, produced by your body. Scientists have identified more than 100 neurotransmitters, and there may be more. Each neurotransmitter carries certain kinds of messages, and each delivers those messages to specific brain cell proteins, called receptors.

Some of these chemical messengers and their adjoining receptors transmit signals to systems in your body that make you feel alert and awake. And some work together to regulate the many important functions and stages of sleep.

In developing medications to promote sleep, scientists uncovered and created other chemicals — substances often produced in a lab — that can interact with these same receptors and alter the messages the receptors receive. In certain instances, the substances make the receptor more sensitive and responsive to the natural neurotransmitter, like turning up the volume on a speaker. In other cases, they may slow or even stop the receptor from receiving the message usually given by the neurotransmitter, like turning down the volume or switching it off altogether.

For more than a century, one neurotransmitter in particular has been of keen interest to researchers who develop sleep medications. Gamma-aminobutyric acid (GABA) is a neurotransmitter with the crucial role of putting the brakes on the body's central nervous system and slowing down its processes, thereby promoting both relaxation and sleep.

In 1864, a scientist named Adolf von Baeyer produced a chemical that inhibited the body's central nervous system. It became the origin of the class of drugs known today as barbiturates. Since then, scientists have determined that what von Baeyer's drug was doing essentially was turning up the volume on the neurotransmitter GABA.

With this effect on GABA, barbiturates acted as tranquilizers that put people to sleep. For the first half of the 20th century, they were commonly used and available worldwide. Americans could buy barbiturates without a prescription, and by the 1940s were consuming more than 1 billion barbiturate pills a year.

But barbiturates also had a significant downside. They were potentially very dangerous and often led to overdoses. That's because these medications weren't selective in their action. They inhibited all parts of the central nervous system, including suppressing breathing. A dose too large could halt breathing altogether. Dependence also became a problem for many people, and withdrawal symptoms could be severe. In the 1950s, Congress stepped in and for the first time required a prescription from a doctor to obtain barbiturates.

At about the same time, researchers discovered another class of chemicals that also acted on the central nervous system. Although they didn't understand it then, these medicines, called benzodiazepines, worked in the same way as barbiturates, by turning up the volume on the GABA neurotransmitter. The big difference, however, was that benzodiazepines were somewhat more selective and didn't suppress breathing as dramatically as did barbiturates, making them potentially less dangerous.

With time, however, dependence and abuse became a growing problem with these medications as well. Use of benzodiazepines — which include the drug diazepam (Valium) — became widespread in the 1960s and '70s, and their abuse became part of popular culture, portrayed in movies and lyricized in songs. Benzodiazepines are still prescribed today, most often to treat anxiety and panic disorders, and less commonly to treat seizures and induce sleep. Their abuse, though relatively rare, remains a problem.

By the 1980s and '90s, scientists were still taking aim at GABA receptors, but with substances other than barbiturates or benzodiazepines. An important group of medications developed around this time is commonly referred to today as non-benzodiazepine benzodiazepine receptor agonists.

These drugs affect GABA receptors in an even more targeted way than previous medications, reducing the undesirable effects of some benzodiazepines. These drugs, which are often referred to as Z-drugs, include medications heavily marketed today: eszopiclone (Lunesta), zaleplon (Sonata) and zolpidem (Ambien, Ambien CR, Edluar).

In the late 1990s, scientists started looking beyond GABA receptors for ways to more safely induce sleep. They discovered the neurotransmitter hypocretin (orexin), involved in the body's sleep-wake cycle and partly responsible for keeping you awake. Researchers found that turning down the volume on orexin helped some people sleep better. This class of medications, known as orexin inhibitors, includes the drugs suvorexant (Belsomra), lemborexant (Dayvigo) and daridorexant (Quviviq).

As these newer drugs were being developed, medications developed for other purposes that also had a sedative effect, such as certain antidepressants, were being prescribed to promote sleep. And nonprescription products, such as herbs and hormones, claiming to induce sleep began to fill store shelves.

A recent report from the Centers for Disease Control and Prevention (CDC) found that approximately 8.4% of U.S. adults today use some type of sleeping medication to help them sleep.

COMMON SLEEP MEDICATIONS

Prescription sleeping pills can help you get to sleep, stay asleep or both. Doctors generally don't recommend relying on prescription sleeping pills for more than a few weeks, but many of these medications are approved for long-term use.

Zolpidem, eszopiclone and zaleplon
This group of medications — the Z-drugs — became widely accepted to treat sleep disorders, including insomnia, following the Food and Drug Administration's approval of zolpidem (Ambien). The Z-drugs include the medications zolpidem (Ambien, Ambien CR, Edluar), eszopiclone (Lunesta) and zaleplon (Sonata).

Zolpidem is the most commonly prescribed medication for the treatment of difficult insomnia. By one analysis, more than 2.5 million people in the United States take zolpidem each year. Because it's metabolized within hours, it also comes in an extended-release form (Ambien CR) designed to produce lasting effects through the night.

The Food and Drug Administration (FDA) recommends that the dose of zolpidem for women be half that for men, based on studies that found higher amounts of the medication in blood tests of women than of men the following morning. However, other studies have questioned this conclusion.

Zaleplon (Sonata) has a shorter half-life than zolpidem, meaning it is eliminated from the body more quickly. For that reason, it's sometimes used by individuals who have trouble going back to sleep after waking in the middle of the night. The opposite is true with eszopiclone (Lunesta), which has a longer half-life and has been associated with a "hangover" effect the next day. Symptoms can include a headache, feeling dehydrated or feeling fatigued or depressed. Eszopiclone also has an unusual side effect where some people complain of a metallic taste in the mouth after taking it.

Each of these medications is approved by the FDA for short-term use; however, in specific circumstances some individuals may benefit from using them for longer periods.

Like their predecessors the benzodiazepines, these medications were developed to promote sleep by slowing parts of the central nervous system. They do this by increasing the effect of the

HOW INSOMNIA MEDICATIONS WORK

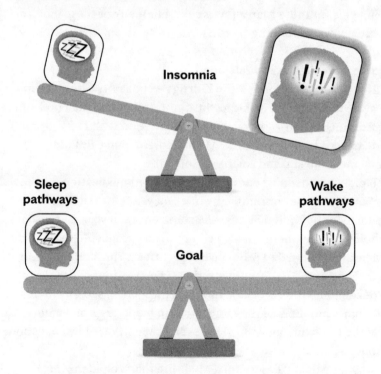

Insomnia medications target overactive pathways. Some enhance sleep pathways, while others inhibit wakefulness pathways, creating better balance between the two.

neurotransmitter GABA and its receptors, resulting in relaxation and sleepiness. Compared with benzodiazepines, these medications are more selective as they attach to receptors, reducing unwanted side effects. They can still produce undesirable effects, however.

Z-drugs have been associated with unusual and potentially dangerous behavior at night, prompting the FDA to require a safety warning in the packaging. Some research suggests an increased risk of having an accident while driving after taking these medications. Other adverse effects can include lasting grogginess, amnesia, abuse, falls, dizziness and cognitive changes.

Z-DRUGS AND UNUSUAL SLEEP BEHAVIORS

Makers of the so-called Z-drugs — eszopiclone (Lunesta), zaleplon (Sonata) and zolpidem (Ambien, Ambien CR, Edluar) — are required by the FDA to warn users about the risk of unusual activities during sleep. Though rare, these "complex sleep behaviors" can be extremely dangerous and can include walking, cooking, eating, having sex, making phone calls or driving while in a sleep state. Usually, the person has no memory of having done this the next day.

This warning included with the medication is the strongest that the FDA can require. It advises anyone who's previously experienced similar behavior during sleep not to take these medications.

Before issuing the warning, the FDA studied records spanning 25 years and found 66 cases that led to serious injury from falls, traffic accidents, drowning, attempted suicide and other incidents. Twenty of the incidents were fatal. Zolpidem was involved in nearly all those cases.

For most people, these widely used medications are safe. However, if you've ever done something during sleep that you don't remember while taking the medication, discuss it with your doctor immediately.

Temazepam

Temazepam (Restoril) is a benzodiazepine and is commonly used to treat insomnia symptoms, helping people fall asleep faster and stay asleep longer. It quickly gained popularity after its approval by the FDA in 1981, and within a decade it accounted for at least 40% of the U.S. market for sleep-inducing medications.

However, the potential for physical dependence and abuse of this drug is relatively high. The body can also become tolerant to the medication, decreasing its effectiveness. For these reasons, and with the emergence of non-benzodiazepine benzodiazepine receptor agonists, use of temazepam has declined. Temazepam is best taken only for a short time, generally 7 to 10 days.

Temazepam works by slowing brain activity. Like the other benzodiazepines, it does this by increasing the effectiveness of the neurotransmitter GABA, which acts as a sedative and inhibits the signaling of neurons. These actions commonly reduce breathing, heart rate and brain activity. The effects can lead to decreased anxiety and sleepiness. While sleepiness might be the desired effect in the evening, it can last into the next day, which is often undesirable and can be dangerous. Benzodiazepines also can change the architecture of sleep, decreasing the amount of restorative deep sleep and rapid eye movement (REM) sleep. Withdrawal symptoms associated with temazepam dependence have been compared to those of alcohol dependence.

Temazepam carries a warning to avoid taking opioid medications at the same time, as this can reduce breathing to a dangerous level and cause death. Also, benzodiazepines shouldn't be taken during pregnancy because of potential harm to the fetus.

Suvorexant, lemborexant and daridorexant

While some medications — including those that target the GABA receptors — work by increasing sleepiness, another strategy to promote sleep takes the opposite approach: These medications instead decrease wakefulness. The difference is more than semantics.

Orexin is a powerful neurotransmitter that your body produces during the day. When it binds with receptors in the nervous system, it makes you feel awake and alert. When the orexin signaling process is disturbed, however, it can lead to narcolepsy, a condition characterized by chronic sleepiness. Without orexin, the body loses some of its ability to stay awake. With this knowledge, researchers explored whether interrupting this chemical messenger could dial down sensations of being wide awake that make it difficult for some people to sleep.

Dual orexin receptor antagonists (DORAs) are a relatively new class of sleep medications that block the action of orexin. These medications, also known as orexin inhibitors, target orexin receptors,

A POTENTIALLY FATAL MIX

Combining sleep medications with opioids can be extremely dangerous, leading to possible overdose and death. Opioids, also known as narcotics, are a class of drugs designed to relieve pain. Both opioids and benzodiazepine medications work in a similar manner — by slowing the body's central nervous system in a way that also reduces breathing.

When sleep medications are taken at the same time as opioids, the combination can lead to coma and death. About 1 in 7 deaths from opioid overdose also involve benzodiazepines.

Prescription medications that contain either benzodiazepines or opioids, such as medications taken for cough or pain, are required by the FDA to include a warning that using the two drugs in combination can suppress breathing and lead to death. The agency has instructed doctors and other medical professionals not to prescribe the two types of medications in combination unless other treatments are inadequate.

More recently, researchers concluded that the combination of opioids and the Z-drugs is also potentially harmful. One study found a substantial increase in the risk of overdose among individuals who were prescribed both an opioid medication and one of the Z-drugs.

turning down the volume on wakefulness. Because their actions are more specific, the drugs don't carry the broader sedating effects of medications such as benzodiazepines and non-benzodiazepines that target GABA receptors. Additionally, orexin inhibitors don't produce withdrawal symptoms and there isn't evidence that you can develop a tolerance to them.

Approved within the last 10 years, these medications include the drugs suvorexant (Belsomra), lemborexant (Dayvigo) and daridorexant (Quviviq). Because daridorexant is processed by the body more quickly than the others, it may be less likely to cause sleepiness the next day.

Ramelteon
This medication takes yet another approach, mimicking the action of the sleep hormone melatonin. Ramelteon (Rozerem) does this by binding with the same receptors in the nervous system as does melatonin, yet it doesn't interact with other parts of the nervous system to induce sedation.

Ramelteon is approved by the FDA for use in helping people fall asleep, but it doesn't increase the total time spent asleep or the amount of time in deep sleep. One thorough review of ramelteon's effectiveness found that it led to improvements in several sleep measures, though the improvements were small. Because of the targeted way it works, it has fewer adverse effects than many other sleep medications.

Trazodone and doxepin
A number of antidepressant medications are also used to treat insomnia. Some have received FDA approval as sleep aids, while others are prescribed off-label to help induce sleep, a common practice. When antidepressants are used solely to treat insomnia, they're typically prescribed before bed and at much lower doses than when taken for other reasons.

Use of antidepressants for treating sleep problems has increased due to concerns associated with abuse of and dependence on benzodiazepines. Trazodone, developed decades ago for the treatment of depression, is commonly prescribed for insomnia. It improves mood by increasing levels of the neurotransmitter serotonin and attaching to receptors for histamine, a substance that causes alertness, among other things. By turning down the volume on the histamine messaging system, trazodone causes drowsiness.

Many medical professionals view trazodone as a good option for some people because the side effects are often more acceptable than those of other sleep medications. However, there isn't universal agreement within the medical field on whether trazodone is suitable as a first-line treatment for insomnia. The American Academy of Sleep Medicine, the American College of Physicians, the U.S. Department of Veterans Affairs and some other medical groups don't recommend prescribing trazodone as a first-line treatment for insomnia. Interestingly, however, trazodone prescriptions for insomnia now exceed the number of prescriptions for depression.

Doxepin (Silenor) is another antidepressant often used for sleep. It has received FDA approval as a treatment for insomnia. When prescribed in low doses, it acts primarily as an antihistamine, which causes drowsiness. Doxepin is typically taken by people who have trouble staying asleep, rather than those who struggle to fall asleep.

OVER-THE-COUNTER SLEEP AIDS

Maybe it's been weeks since you've had a good night's sleep. You haven't seen a doctor about your sleep troubles, and now you're wondering if maybe you should just try a nonprescription sleep aid and see what happens. If you're considering an over-the-counter medication to help you sleep, here are some things you should know.

Most sleep aids available without a prescription contain antihistamines. Tolerance to the sedative effects of antihistamines can develop quickly. So, the longer you take them, the less likely they are to make you sleepy.

In addition, some sleep aids available without a prescription can leave you feeling groggy and unwell the next day. This is the so-called hangover effect. Medication interactions are possible as well, and much remains unknown about the safety and effectiveness of sleep aids available without a prescription.

Nonprescription products to help you sleep are widely available. The following are the most commonly used sleep aids.

Antihistamine products

Many over-the-counter sleep aids — products such as ZzzQuil and Unisom — contain antihistamines. Antihistamines were developed to make people with allergies feel more comfortable by drying up runny noses and watery eyes. But they also carry a significant side effect: They make you drowsy.

Nonprescription antihistamine-based sleep products are widely advertised. And people hoping for a good night's sleep spend billions

MEDICATION RECOMMENDATIONS

In its guidelines for medical professionals who prescribe drugs, the American Academy of Sleep Medicine makes recommendations regarding use of more than a dozen sleep medications and sleep aids. These recommendations are based on the organization's standards and the available evidence at the time and are compared against providing no treatment. Here are the organization's recommendations regarding currently used sleep medicines.

Medication	Treatment goal	Recommendation
Doxepin	Staying asleep	Recommend
Eszopiclone	Falling asleep, staying asleep	Recommend
Ramelteon	Falling asleep	Recommend
Suvorexant	Staying asleep	Recommend
Temazepam	Falling asleep, staying asleep	Recommend

of dollars on them each year. However, despite their popularity, over-the-counter sleep aids are generally poor at providing long-term relief from insomnia symptoms and have some potential downsides.

When used to promote sleep, the sleepiness produced by antihistamines is desirable, whereas the drying of the nose and sinuses isn't. Also, the medications can cause lingering drowsiness that can carry over to the next day. And they can cause dizziness. That, combined with hangover effects from the drugs, can lead to falls. Other side effects may include daytime constipation and urinary retention. Certain antihistamines also have been associated with cognitive impairment and increased risk of dementia, especially among older people.

Triazolam	Falling asleep	Recommend
Zaleplon	Falling asleep	Recommend
Zolpidem	Falling asleep, staying asleep	Recommend
Diphenhydramine	Falling asleep, staying asleep	Don't recommend
Melatonin	Falling asleep, staying asleep	Don't recommend
Tiagabine	Falling asleep, staying asleep	Don't recommend
Trazodone	Falling asleep, staying asleep	Don't recommend
Tryptophan	Falling asleep, staying asleep	Don't recommend
Valerian	Falling asleep, staying asleep	Don't recommend

WHAT TO LOOK FOR

Pharmacy and grocery store aisles are packed with supplements and other over-the-counter products with nuanced claims suggesting they can help you sleep. Some of the substances in the bottles were identified centuries ago and are still around, while others were developed in modern labs. With their promise of "supporting" or "promoting" sleep, these products can be very alluring. For most people, however, that promise is never realized.

For many supplements, the research doesn't show them to be effective for treating sleep disorders. Often, any positive results that people do experience are small.

It's important to remember that supplements aren't regulated with the same strict quality control requirements that apply to medications. Studies also show that contamination and inaccurate dosages are common with supplements.

If you use supplements, a couple of things can help ensure you're getting what you think you are, and that the product meets some nongovernment standards. Look for labels that contain the following:

- **USP Verified.** This indicates that the supplement has been independently tested and meets standards set by United States Pharmacopeia, a nonprofit organization.
- **GMP.** This attests that the product meets standards for good manufacturing practices, set by NSF, an independent organization formerly known as the National Sanitation Foundation.

If you try supplements, note when you begin taking them, and pay close attention to whether the supplement is having the effect you want. Are you sleeping better at night? Do you have more energy during the day? If you find after a time that you're not getting the desired results, it's best to stop using the product. Stop immediately if you notice any undesirable side effects.

In addition, though antihistamines aren't habit-forming, your body quickly becomes used to them and they become less effective. One study found it took just three days of use for one type of antihistamine to lose its effectiveness.

Some prominent physician groups recommend against the use of antihistamines for help falling asleep and staying asleep. They say research shows that antihistamines don't significantly help people sleep.

Melatonin

The popularity of melatonin supplements has exploded over the years, with millions of people using them for a variety of sleep disorders, including management of jet lag and reducing the time it takes to fall asleep. Melatonin is generally considered safe and has been shown to produce modest benefits, but the many unknowns about its long-term use raise questions and concerns. Also, quality control has been a problem for as long as melatonin has been sold, leading to contamination and inaccurate dosages in many products.

Melatonin is a natural hormone important to your natural sleep-wake cycle. The pineal gland in your brain produces melatonin at the direction of the brain control center responsible for the body's circadian rhythms (see page 57). During the day, melatonin levels naturally dip in response to light. At night, they rise in preparation for sleep. Your body makes only a tiny amount of melatonin, about one-tenth of a milligram (mg). The quantity of melatonin you produce decreases as you grow older, which may affect how well you sleep.

Melatonin available in stores or sold online is similar to the natural hormone, but the supplement is most likely made in a lab (although it can also be produced by microorganisms or animals). Melatonin supplements are often taken in doses of 2 or 5 mg, which is many times higher than the amount your body naturally produces. This is in part because your body can't absorb or use much of the melatonin you take orally.

Studies show that melatonin supplements may produce modest benefits for treating insomnia. One well-known study found that using melatonin reduced the time it takes to fall asleep by 4 minutes and increased the total time asleep by almost 13 minutes. These modest results are consistent with labeling on some melatonin bottles, such as: "SLEEP * Fall Asleep Faster * Stay Asleep Longer."

When the FDA first approved the sale of melatonin, the agency regulated the synthetic hormone as a dietary supplement, not as a medication. That meant it wasn't evaluated for its medical benefits or potential harm. Researchers warn that despite its popularity, long-term melatonin use hasn't been well studied. Generally, however, it's considered safe when compared to prescription or other over-the-counter sleep medications.

The American Academy of Sleep Medicine recommends against using melatonin to treat insomnia symptoms. The organization states that studies indicating melatonin helped people to sleep could be flawed, and reliable research suggests the supplement didn't improve sleep by much.

BE WARY OF MELATONIN LABELS

The bottle in the supplement aisle at your local pharmacy may say that each melatonin tablet contains 2 mg of melatonin, but there's a good chance it actually will deliver a very different dose. Labels on melatonin supplements are commonly inaccurate, raising important safety questions.

One recent study analyzed 25 brands of melatonin gummies sold in the United States and found that only three were within 10% of what was printed on the bottle. The other 22 contained from 74% to 347% of what the manufacturer claimed. Previous studies had found some melatonin doses nearly five times higher than expected, and some also contained serotonin, a controlled substance.

Because federal regulators consider melatonin a supplement, the FDA does not hold it to the same quality standards as medications. If you buy melatonin, look for labels that have USP Verified or GMP (good manufacturing practice) logos, which show the product meets quality standards for supplements.

If you believe that melatonin is helpful to your sleep, it's probably OK to keep using it. It's best to take it about 30 minutes prior to bedtime, and not to exceed 10 mg.

Melatonin and jet lag

While long-distance air travel puts you in a new destination, your circadian rhythms are likely staying put in the place you left. This can cause jet lag, making you sleepy when you want to be alert and frustratingly wide awake when you want to sleep. Jet lag can cause short-term disruption to your sleep, often when you want to be in top form for work or alert while on vacation.

Use of melatonin is commonly accepted as a short-term treatment for jet lag, helping to reset your body's internal clock. Timing is important, though. After flying east, take melatonin at the local bedtime. When flying west, take it in the morning until you adjust to the new time zone. A dose of 0.5 mg is typically as effective as larger amounts.

Also, if you're tired while traveling, it may not be jet lag. When crossing three or fewer time zones, you may just be fatigued rather than jet-lagged.

Gamma-aminobutyric acid (GABA)

Gamma-aminobutyric acid is an amino acid found in plants, animals and even bacteria and fungi. It's also a brain neurotransmitter responsible for slowing down the nervous system to help calm and relax you.

Many people eat GABA-rich foods or take it as a supplement with the aim of improving their sleep. Some foods naturally contain GABA in greater amounts, including tea, tomatoes and soybeans. Manufactured GABA is often produced by microbial fermentation.

However, questions remain about how much, if any, of the GABA you swallow makes it through the blood-brain barrier that keeps many substances in your blood out of the brain. According to one review of the research, studies offer "very limited evidence" that GABA taken orally improves sleep.

Cannabis

The cannabis industry has surged since California voters first approved cannabis for medical use in 1996. Since then, many states and the District of Columbia have introduced medical cannabis programs, often also allowing nonmedical cannabis use among adults.

Surveys show that trouble sleeping is one of the most common reasons people cite for using cannabis. In fact, some studies indicate that the use of sleep medications has dropped in places where cannabis has become legally available.

Despite this widespread acceptance, the science doesn't support cannabis as an effective treatment for insomnia and other sleep disorders. A recent review of five decades of research on cannabis and sleep found cannabis worsened sleep rather than improved it in most studies.

The cannabis plant produces several chemicals that interact with the neurological signaling system that controls some of the most important processes in your body. Two of those chemicals, cannabidiol (CBD) and delta-9-tetrahydrocannabinol (THC), are particularly potent, with THC being responsible for making people feel high. Some researchers believe that these and many other compounds in the cannabis plant hold promise for helping people sleep, but other scientists say not enough research has been done to support that conclusion.

Studies involving cannabis have been slowed because the FDA long classified it as a Schedule I drug, along with substances such as heroin and LSD. Also because of the Schedule I classification, there was no federal oversight of state cannabis programs and none of the basic science that regulators require for medical use of a substance. States approved cannabis programs in defiance of the federal position, and this has led to a patchwork of laws and standards.

Because cannabis hasn't received the research attention it warrants, it's not possible to definitively answer some of the most basic, important questions about cannabis and sleep. High-quality studies involving the use of cannabis products by people with insomnia and other disorders are few and far between, and they show mixed results. A study of people with insomnia and anxiety showed that after two months of using CBD, 56% had improved sleep, but nearly 27% reported worse sleep.

Cannabis also has several negative effects, especially for adolescents and young adults. Among other things, it can impair driving and lead to daytime sleepiness. And cannabis users trying to quit often experience withdrawal symptoms that can include disrupted sleep.

Talk to your doctor before using cannabis to help you sleep.

Herbal supplements

Perhaps you've heard or read that some herbal supplements help promote sleep. For the most part, herbal products haven't been shown to improve sleep, and some can even be dangerous.

Valerian

Valerian, a flowering perennial plant sometimes called all-heal, has been used as an herbal remedy since ancient times and is now widely sold with vague claims suggesting that it can help ease anxiety and reduce insomnia. Scientific support, however, is inconclusive.

There are more than 200 species of valerian, though *Valeriana officinalis* is the one most commonly found in supplements. A native of Europe and Asia, it now grows wild in the United States. The plant's roots and stems are dried to produce supplements in capsule form, as well as a tea or tincture.

Researchers have isolated a myriad of chemical compounds in valerian but have been unable to determine which might promote sleep. And a comprehensive review of the available research found inconsistent results that valerian can treat insomnia symptoms. One randomized, placebo-controlled trial, the gold standard in research, failed to find that valerian improved sleep among people undergoing cancer treatment.

Valerian is considered safe for most individuals but can cause nausea and abdominal cramps in some. Risks to children and to pregnant individuals or those who are nursing haven't been studied.

Kava

A pepper plant native to the West Pacific, kava has been used for thousands of years and is now sold as a supplement for anxiety and insomnia.

While research has shown that kava may have a small effect on anxiety, there's been less study of its impact on sleep. A number of active compounds unique to the plant have been identified, yet researchers don't have a clear understanding of how they contribute to a feeling of relaxation.

Because kava has been associated with liver injury, which in some cases has been fatal, it should be avoided as a sleep aid. It also can produce other side effects including headaches, fatigue and restlessness. Some researchers have raised concerns about quality control and the safety of processes used to produce the capsule form.

Jujube seed
With a long history in traditional Chinese medicine, jujube seed remains popular today for people seeking to relieve anxiety. It's also reputed to have sleep-inducing effects. Researchers have shown that compounds in the plant interact with the same GABA messaging system in the brain that some prescription sleep medications target.

Studies done in rats have shown an increase in sleep, but studies on humans aren't widely available. The product is generally considered to be safe.

USE SLEEP MEDICATIONS WISELY

As mentioned earlier in this chapter and in the previous chapter, sleeping pills may help when stress, travel or other disruptions keep you awake. For long-term insomnia, behavior changes learned in cognitive behavioral therapy for insomnia (CBT-I) are usually the best treatment.

Prescription sleeping pills, and even some nonprescription sleeping aids, as well as certain antidepressants, may not be safe if you're pregnant, breastfeeding or an older adult. Among older adults, sleeping pills can increase the risk of nighttime falls and injury. Also, having certain health conditions — for example, kidney disease, low blood pressure, heart rhythm problems or a history of seizures — may limit your medication options.

If you take other medications, prescription or over-the-counter, keep in mind that sleeping pills may interact with them. So, it's very important to talk with your doctor before adding another drug to the mix.

If you do take sleep medication or an over-the-counter sleep aid, here are some tips on how to take the product safely:

- **Get a medical evaluation.** See your primary care provider for a thorough exam before taking a nonprescription product, as well as a prescription drug. If you're taking sleeping pills for more than a few weeks, ask about an appropriate follow-up schedule to discuss if the medicines are working.
- **Read the medication guide.** Make sure you understand how and when to take your medicine and what the major potential side effects are. If you have any questions, ask your pharmacist or someone on your healthcare team.
- **Never take a sleeping pill until you're going to bed.** Sleeping pills can make you less aware of what you're doing, increasing the risk of dangerous situations. Wait to take your sleeping pill until you've completed all your evening activities, and right before you plan on sleeping.
- **Watch for side effects.** If you feel sleepy or dizzy during the day or if you experience any other side effects that bother you, see your doctor, who may suggest trying a different medicine, changing your dose or weaning you off the pills.
- **Avoid alcohol.** Never mix alcohol and sleeping pills. Alcohol increases the sedative effects of the pills. Even a small amount of alcohol combined with sleeping pills can make you feel dizzy, confused or faint. Combining alcohol with certain sleeping pills can lead to dangerously slowed breathing or unresponsiveness. And alcohol itself can cause insomnia.
- **Don't take sleeping pills with opioids.** Opioids include pain-relieving prescription medicines such as oxycodone, hydrocodone, morphine, methadone and the synthetic opioid fentanyl. The drug class also includes illegal drugs, such as heroin. Combining an opioid with sleeping pills can be dangerous. The combination increases the sedative effects of the pills and can lead to slowed breathing or unresponsiveness. It can even cause you to stop breathing.
- **Take the medications strictly as prescribed.** Take only the amount prescribed. If the initial dose doesn't produce the intended effect on sleep, don't take more pills without first talking to your doctor.

- **Quit carefully.** When you're ready to stop taking sleeping pills, follow instructions from your doctor or pharmacist or the directions on the label. Some medicines must be stopped gradually. Also, be aware that you may have some short-term rebound insomnia for a few days after you stop taking sleeping pills.

8

Sleep apnea

John was in his cardiologist's office to discuss his high blood pressure when the doctor asked him a seemingly random question: Do you snore?

In fact, John did snore while sleeping. It sometimes woke him up, and his wife certainly reminded him about it often enough. Snoring is a common symptom of sleep apnea, which can increase the risk of high blood pressure. "I think [my cardiologist] thought there might be a connection," said John.

John took an overnight sleep test, giving him a definitive diagnosis of obstructive sleep apnea. The results of that test were dramatic: He averaged 52 breathing disruptions per hour, well above the threshold for severe apnea of 30 disruptions per hour. His blood oxygen levels had dipped as low as 82% during the night; values under 90% are considered low.

"I was surprised," John said. "I guess I didn't know what a good night's sleep was."

The doctor at the sleep clinic prescribed a continuous positive airway pressure (CPAP) device, which delivers air pressure through a mask while you sleep. John got the equipment right away and began to use it.

The benefits weren't immediate, however. Like many, he struggled with some of the realities of CPAP. In the five years he has been using the treatment, he's switched mask styles several times, always looking for the most comfortable one. Some masks rubbed on his skin and left a mark — "CPAP nose," he calls it. He believes he still hasn't found that perfect mask.

But despite these rough spots, he's a firm believer in CPAP and sees how it has helped him. He now averages about five apnea events per hour, a tiny fraction of what he experienced during his sleep test.

"My wife says I have a lot more energy now that I use the CPAP," John said. "I feel a lot more rested when I get up. I do feel better."

John has taken other steps, too, as part of an overall approach to improving his sleep. He has lost about 50 pounds after learning that being overweight contributes to obstructive sleep apnea. He's also tried to improve his sleep generally by sticking to a regular sleep schedule, going to bed and waking at about the same time every day.

John credits these things, along with his medications, for lowering his blood pressure significantly and improving his health, and for making him feel more vigorous during the day.

"If you don't sleep well, that affects a lot of things mentally and physically," he said. "So I focus on getting better sleep."

Perhaps you frequently wake in the night, gasping for breath. Or maybe you've been told that you snore loudly, and during the day you lack energy and the ability to concentrate. Signs like these may leave you wondering whether you have obstructive sleep apnea, a potentially serious condition that can harm your overall health and well-being.

Obstructive sleep apnea is a breathing disorder that starves your body of oxygen and prevents you from getting a good night's sleep. During sleep, the soft tissue in your throat and air passage can collapse, blocking you from taking a breath until you wake up at least enough for the airway to reopen, allowing you to breathe again. This can happen dozens of times each hour, well over 100 times in a night.

Your risk of developing obstructive sleep apnea increases with age and excess weight, and Americans are getting both older and heavier. Aging baby boomers have pushed the median age to nearly 40 and obesity rates have soared, reaching more than 40% this century. As more people become at risk, it's not surprising that there's a growing awareness of obstructive sleep apnea.

Obstructive sleep apnea is relatively common, affecting 14% of men and 5% of women in the United States. A similar condition, called central sleep apnea, occurs when the signaling between the lungs and the brain breaks down during sleep and leads to disruptions in breathing. This condition isn't nearly as common as obstructive sleep apnea, and by one estimate it affects less than 1% of U.S. adults. Central sleep apnea is discussed later in this chapter.

Sleep apnea can take a heavy toll on your overall health and how you feel each day. Having sleep apnea increases your risk of several serious medical conditions, including high blood pressure, type 2 diabetes and stroke. Quality of life usually suffers as well.

One risk deserves special attention. If you have obstructive sleep apnea, you're at significantly increased risk of having a motor vehicle accident. Driving while drowsy puts both you and others in danger. This risk is increased further with use of alcohol and medications that have a sedative effect.

Fortunately, sleep apnea is often highly treatable with ongoing therapy. Disruptions to breathing and sleep associated with the condition can be greatly reduced or eliminated altogether. Many people refer to the treatments as life-changing or even lifesaving. Treatments range from weight loss to devices that apply constant pressure to your airway, and from mouthpieces that nudge your jaw open just a bit to sophisticated electronics that influence the position in which you sleep.

In this chapter you'll learn what causes sleep apnea and how it's diagnosed. In the next chapter we explain how sleep apnea is treated. We'll provide practical tips, based on decades of experience treating individuals with sleep apnea, about ways to improve your chances of successful treatment and return to nights of restorative sleep. We've seen the benefits of treatment up close and believe you can experience them as well.

BREATH OF LIFE

Breathing seems so simple and uncomplicated that a person hardly ever thinks about it. In fact, it's an elaborately choreographed sequence of actions in the body, regulated by a vast network of neurons in a part of the brain that controls basic, vital functions.

Each breath starts at the nostrils or mouth, then makes the short journey through the airway, passing through your throat (pharynx), voice box (larynx), and windpipe (trachea) and into the bronchial tubes in the lungs. When the air reaches your lungs, it flows into about 150 million minuscule air sacs (alveoli). These air sacs are densely lined with capillaries, small blood vessels with such thin walls that oxygen can pass through them to enter your bloodstream. There, the oxygen courses through your body to feed your cells so they can do their work.

When you exhale, you rid your body of some carbon dioxide, a waste product of all that cellular activity.

Your breathing constantly adapts throughout your waking day, growing faster and deeper to deliver more oxygen and remove more carbon dioxide when you're active, and then slowing when you're still. This rhythm is regulated by sensors in the brain and blood vessels that closely track how much oxygen is in your blood and the acidity that carbon dioxide creates.

The mechanics of apnea

As you fall asleep each night, your breathing patterns change. Because you're resting, breathing can slow, and during some sleep stages it grows shallow. Even during healthy sleep, carbon dioxide levels in the blood typically rise just a bit.

The muscles in your body — including in your throat — cycle through varying levels of relaxation during a night's sleep. When muscles in your tongue and throat relax, the opening in your airway can shrink, increasing air resistance. In some people, the airway narrows to the size of a drinking straw. As air passes through this constricted opening, it roils with turbulence and can vibrate the soft tissues in the throat, creating the familiar sounds of snoring. Sleeping on your back can add to the problem as the tug of gravity pulls down the tongue and other tissues, making the throat more susceptible to collapse.

When the airway narrows all the way and no air can reach the lungs, it's called apnea. When the blockage reduces airflow by at least 30%, enough to cause a drop in oxygen or to interrupt sleep, the condition is known as hypopnea. Both are serious.

During these breathing disruptions, oxygen levels plunge by as much as 40%, carbon dioxide levels rise, and your blood becomes more acidic. Sensors in your brain stem and elsewhere detect this and send an urgent SOS signal to wake you. As your body rouses you from sleep, your muscle tone returns, opening your airway and allowing normal breathing to resume. All this may happen repeatedly, though you may never wake up enough to become aware of it.

Breathing disruptions don't necessarily happen throughout the entire night. The extent to which your muscles relax changes during the different stages of sleep. Your muscles are most relaxed during rapid eye movement (REM) sleep, when you lose some of your ability to move, preventing you from acting out your dreams. Because this also affects the muscles in the throat, REM sleep can be the most likely time to experience complete closure of the airway. Breathing disruptions, however, can create apnea episodes during any phase of sleep. Light sleep, too, can be a period of unstable breathing for some.

These constant disruptions to your sleep can upset your body's ability to cycle through the different stages of sleep. Ideally, you should pass from light sleep to deeper sleep, and then to REM sleep, before going back to light sleep. This sequence happens many times each night. With sleep apnea, however, it's easy to get stuck in light sleep. Breathing disruptions awaken you while you're still in light sleep, and you then fall back into light sleep, only to be repeatedly roused again. Your body is cheated of the deep, restorative sleep that's so important to your long-term health and to how you feel each day.

Waking repeatedly also creates a cascading effect on your body's stress systems. Your body responds to the lack of oxygen and excess carbon dioxide by activating its fight-or-flight response, releasing stress hormones such as adrenaline and norepinephrine. These hormones increase your heart rate, blood pressure and overall metabolic rate, preparing you to respond to a perceived threat. When this happens repeatedly, it takes a toll on your heart and blood vessels, leading to problems such as high blood pressure, heart disease, atrial

NORMAL VS. OBSTRUCTED BREATHING

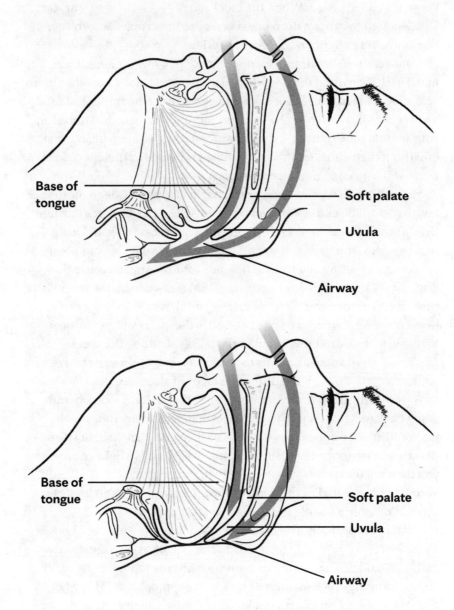

The top image shows normal breathing while sleeping. The bottom image shows obstructive sleep apnea. Notice how muscles in the tongue and throat relax, blocking the flow of air into the lungs.

fibrillation or stroke. Plus, it means that you don't sleep well, making you feel tired during the day.

Some people find it difficult to fall back asleep after waking. Sleep apnea can contribute to insomnia, even when it's relatively mild. The repeated adrenaline rush and fight-or-flight response make it difficult to get deep, restful sleep. If you're also experiencing insomnia, you might find it hard to fall asleep or stay asleep, or you may wake up too early and not be able to go back to sleep. Poor sleep only makes the body more stressed, creating a cycle of sleep problems.

In rare instances, disturbed sleep patterns caused by apnea episodes can trigger unusual sleep-related behaviors such as sleepwalking or acting out dreams. Some people with apnea start to grind their teeth during sleep.

CAUSES AND RISK FACTORS

Millions of people are at increased risk for obstructive sleep apnea. Your throat and upper airway anatomy, along with your overall health and lifestyle, can make it more likely that your airway will narrow during sleep. Your gender and age are factors as well. Obstructive sleep apnea occurs up to three times more frequently among men than among women. However, the likelihood for both increases with age.

Excess weight
Being overweight is the most important risk factor. People who are significantly overweight are extremely likely to have obstructive sleep apnea. A 10% weight gain has been shown to cause a sixfold increase in your risk of developing moderate to severe obstructive sleep apnea.

Excess weight triggers several physical and hormonal changes that affect breathing during sleep. Body fat develops within the tongue and throat, causing the airway to narrow and making it more likely to collapse. Belly fat can push on the diaphragm during sleep, reducing lung capacity. And having large amounts of fat tissue affects levels of leptin, a hormone best known for driving hunger, but which also acts as a breathing stimulant.

Oral anatomy
You're also more likely to experience disrupted breathing during sleep if your lower jaw is short compared to your upper jaw. The shape of the inside of your mouth and throat, as well as the size of your tongue and tonsils, can increase your risk, too. Because these physical traits are determined by genetics, obstructive sleep apnea can be inherited.

Lifestyle
Specific habits, including drinking alcohol and smoking, can contribute to obstructive sleep apnea. Alcohol relaxes the muscles in the throat, making it more likely the airway will collapse. Smoking can cause inflammation that constricts the airway. Some studies suggest that too much caffeine may increase disordered breathing.

OBSTRUCTIVE SLEEP APNEA, OBESITY AND APPETITE

Breathing disruptions that interfere with sleep can upset the balance of two hormones that regulate appetite and weight, called ghrelin and leptin. Ghrelin signals the brain that you're hungry. Leptin makes you feel full and satisfied after eating.

Obesity and obstructive sleep apnea can lead to something called leptin resistance, in which the body doesn't respond to the hormone's signals.

Because of leptin resistance, the brain may not get the message that the body has enough energy stored in the form of fat. This can lead to increased food intake, even though the body has more than enough energy stored.

As you gain weight, sleep apnea can worsen, producing even more disrupted sleep. This creates a cycle: Poor sleep leads to hormonal changes, which bring weight gain, which makes sleep apnea worse, causing poor sleep.

Managing sleep apnea can help break this cycle.

Health

Obstructive sleep apnea is more likely in people with certain serious health conditions, including high blood pressure, diabetes, cardiovascular disease and stroke.

Men vs. women

Men are much more likely to have sleep apnea than are women. Although this gap narrows with age, when women are more likely to

---

OBESITY HYPOVENTILATION SYNDROME

In addition to increased risk of obstructive sleep apnea, people with a body mass index above 30 are at risk of obesity hypoventilation syndrome, which causes poor breathing, lower blood oxygen and increased blood carbon dioxide levels.

Most people with obesity hypoventilation syndrome have symptoms that overlap with obstructive sleep apnea, but they tend to have more persistent daytime sleepiness despite seemingly adequate sleep. They also may have chronic and unexplained shortness of breath during the day and frequent morning headaches. Unlike with sleep apnea, symptoms don't occur only during sleep.

Symptoms associated with obesity hypoventilation syndrome arise because the body isn't able to breathe deeply or effectively enough, causing an imbalance in blood oxygen and carbon dioxide levels. This can cause strain on the heart and symptoms such as swollen legs and shortness of breath. Some people can have difficulties performing day-to-day activities and can even end up in the emergency room.

Treatment for obesity hypoventilation syndrome includes weight loss and breathing assistance, which may include use of a positive airway pressure device worn at night, similar to treatment of obstructive sleep apnea.

develop the condition, it remains much more prevalent in men throughout life.

The way weight is distributed in men compared to women may play a role. The distribution of body fat associated with obesity seems to have a greater impact on the airway of men than of women.

Women are also less likely to be diagnosed with sleep apnea. This may be because their snoring isn't noticed as frequently by their partner, they're less likely to complain about symptoms, or their symptoms are wrongly attributed to insomnia or depression. Also, the fact that sleep apnea is much more common in men has led some to incorrectly think of it as a "men's disease." This bias makes it even more important that women and their partners pay close attention to the warning signs of obstructive sleep apnea and discuss any concerns with a doctor.

Symptoms can also differ between men and women. Women tend to have fewer and shorter breathing disruptions, and more of these are clustered in REM sleep. Also, in women, a smaller percentage of apnea episodes is associated with sleeping on the back.

Obstructive sleep apnea in women becomes more common with the onset of menopause. Women are 3.5 times more likely to have obstructive sleep apnea after menopause than before it. The hormones estrogen and progesterone are believed to offer some protection for women from breathing problems during sleep for much of their lives. When these hormones decrease in menopause, women are more likely to snore and develop obstructive sleep apnea. Hormone replacement therapy hasn't been shown to reverse obstructive sleep apnea.

THE DANGERS OF OBSTRUCTIVE SLEEP APNEA

The tired, fatigued feeling that often accompanies obstructive sleep apnea is reason enough to address it. But the stakes are much higher than that. By stealing both sleep and oxygen from your body, the condition is associated with a wide range of serious health conditions that can detract from your quality of life and even your longevity. Here is how obstructive sleep apnea works to undermine your health in specific ways and how it may be related to other serious health conditions.

High blood pressure
Obstructive sleep apnea can cause high blood pressure (hypertension), a dangerous condition with widespread negative effects on your health. Obstructive sleep apnea can make it four times more likely that you'll experience uncontrolled high blood pressure. The more apnea events you have each night, the greater the odds.

Nearly 1 in 3 people with high blood pressure have obstructive sleep apnea. The numbers soar to 8 out of 10 among people with high blood pressure resistant to medication. One reason for this could be that obstructive sleep apnea makes medication less effective.

High blood pressure is a subtle, sneaky condition, sometimes called the silent killer because it displays no symptoms. As it goes unnoticed, it can cause serious damage to your organs, including your heart, brain, kidneys and eyes. It can contribute to clogging or bursting of the arteries in the brain, causing a stroke. High blood pressure decreases the amount of blood and oxygen that gets to your heart, which can cause cardiovascular disease. Years of untreated high blood pressure can make dementia more likely later in life.

Sleep apnea often causes high blood pressure because of the way it affects oxygen levels and the body's nervous system. When you stop breathing during sleep, your blood becomes starved of oxygen, each time doing a little bit of damage to the tissues within your vascular system. Disrupted sleep also can produce changes to your nervous system, affecting your blood pressure.

Treating obstructive sleep apnea with positive airway pressure therapy is one way to reduce high blood pressure and its negative health outcomes. Many studies have shown both short- and long-term decreases in blood pressure among people who regularly use their positive airway pressure (PAP) devices. (PAP devices are discussed in detail in the next chapter.) This form of treatment may have the greatest impact on individuals whose high blood pressure hasn't been lowered with medication.

Not all experts agree, though, that PAP devices to treat sleep apnea are an effective treatment for reducing high blood pressure. Treatment guidelines developed by the American College of Cardiology and the American Heart Association say that the effectiveness of positive airway pressure on lowering blood pressure is "not well established."

If you have high blood pressure, your treatment may include other therapies, such as medication. Positive airway pressure, however, is an important part of staying healthy.

Diabetes and insulin resistance
Type 2 diabetes is a serious condition in which your blood retains harmful levels of glucose, the sugar that your cells use for energy. This can happen when cells become less sensitive to insulin, the hormone that allows the body to use glucose, so the sugar remains unused in your blood.

Type 2 diabetes and obstructive sleep apnea are closely associated with each other, meaning that a person with one of these conditions has an increased likelihood of having the other. Nearly 3 out of every 4 people who have type 2 diabetes meet the criteria for obesity and have obstructive sleep apnea.

Obstructive sleep apnea affects your body in several ways that could contribute to diabetes. Fragmented sleep and a reduction in oxygen caused by obstructive sleep apnea places stress on the body and alters certain hormones. Some of these hormonal changes can lead to the accumulation of fat, raising the risk of diabetes. Oxygen starvation also can alter your body's response to the hormone insulin, a condition known as insulin resistance, one of the mechanisms associated with type 2 diabetes. Poor sleep on its own is a risk factor for diabetes, too.

It remains unclear whether treatment for sleep apnea improves diabetes. Researchers have noted some promising study results, especially among people who use PAP devices to maintain air pressure for long periods each night. Even if the treatment doesn't immediately reverse the metabolic issues underlying type 2 diabetes, the other health benefits it provides can be especially important.

If you have type 2 diabetes, discuss with your doctor whether you should be evaluated for obstructive sleep apnea, even if you have few or no symptoms.

Stroke
Obstructive sleep apnea can be a risk factor for stroke or occur as a result of one.

Repeated stress on the body from being deprived of oxygen results in high blood pressure and can increase activity of those components in blood responsible for clotting (coagulation). A stroke often results from a clot blocking blood flow to the brain. Obstructive sleep apnea also produces inflammation, which can contribute to stroke. Some people learn they have sleep apnea only after a stroke.

Obstructive sleep apnea also may occur as a consequence of a stroke. Up to 70% of people who've had a stroke have obstructive sleep apnea, and up to 24% have central sleep apnea, a related condition in which the brain's signaling system that tells you when to breathe becomes disrupted. Central sleep apnea may occur as a result of a stroke that involves a part of the brain stem or a bilateral hemispheric stroke, which affects both sides of the brain.

Treatment of obstructive sleep apnea reduces the risk of having a stroke. In one study, risk of stroke decreased by 2% for every month a person used a PAP device over a two-year period. Treatment also decreases the risk of having another stroke. Use of a PAP device after a stroke can lower blood pressure at night and improve attention and neurological recovery, and it can reduce the length of your hospital stay by up to two weeks.

Accidents

Driving a vehicle requires concentration, alertness, good judgment and sound physical performance — qualities that suffer when you're deprived of sleep. Someone with obstructive sleep apnea is at least 2.5 times more likely to have an automobile accident, and the chance of having an accident at work doubles.

One study determined that 800,000 vehicle crashes each year could be attributed to sleep apnea, taking 1,400 lives and costing $15.9 billion. The researchers concluded that proper treatment could save nearly 1,000 lives a year just by reducing crashes.

Strong evidence that obstructive sleep apnea contributes to an increase in accidents has led to calls for screening professional drivers for the condition. When compared to the general population, professional drivers are more likely to have obstructive sleep apnea, in part because a high percentage are overweight, male and middle-aged — three risk factors for the condition.

Daytime sleepiness

A common telltale sign of obstructive sleep apnea is a pervasive feeling of sleepiness that follows you throughout the day. About half of people with obstructive sleep apnea complain of excessive daytime sleepiness, while many others don't feel sleepy during the day at all. This remains one of the ongoing mysteries of obstructive sleep apnea and why it can be difficult to detect.

Sleepiness associated with obstructive sleep apnea results from less time spent in deep, restorative sleep. Sleep deprivation also leads to an increase in levels of cytokines, proteins involved in inflammation. Cytokines make you feel sleepy and put you at risk for developing other health conditions.

Among some people, treating obstructive sleep apnea reduces sleep disruptions but for some reason doesn't lead to a corresponding decrease in sleepiness during the day. It may be possible that oxygen deprivation has injured or destroyed the nerve cells that promote wakefulness. For these individuals, medications that increase daytime wakefulness may be helpful.

Insomnia

Some people have trouble trying to determine which condition they have: sleep apnea or insomnia. In many cases they have both. This is known as comorbid insomnia and sleep apnea (COMISA). Studies suggest that 40% to 60% of people with obstructive sleep apnea also have insomnia.

Sleep apnea can contribute to insomnia in several ways, including the constant, repeated release of stress hormones as your body reacts to the breathing disruptions. Studies suggest that when the two conditions appear simultaneously, there's a higher rate of heart disease.

If you believe you may have both insomnia and obstructive sleep apnea, discuss it with your doctor.

Nighttime urination

Many people find they need to make more trips to the bathroom as they grow older. Needing to use the bathroom more than twice each night is considered excessive nighttime urination, or nocturia. Among men, this is frequently attributed to an enlarged prostate gland, a common occurrence with aging. In women, it's sometimes linked to the increased urine production and reduced bladder size that can come with aging.

Nocturia is also a symptom of obstructive sleep apnea. Sleep apnea causes an increase in the hormones that stimulate urination, and it can increase abdominal pressure. Approximately 70% of people with obstructive sleep apnea have nocturia.

Treatment of sleep apnea may help normalize the imbalance of hormones involved in regulating urination. One analysis found that people using a PAP device to treat their sleep apnea reduced the average number of nightly trips to the bathroom by more than two. However, the effects of treatment on nighttime urination frequency can vary. Some people may experience significant improvements, while others may see only modest changes.

Death
Mortality is a key factor that researchers use to help understand the broad health implications of any condition. Studies show that people with obstructive sleep apnea have an increased risk of death from any cause, and it generally increases with the severity of the condition.

One well-known study found that people with untreated severe obstructive sleep apnea were nearly four times more likely to die than those without the condition. Another study found the risk of death from moderate obstructive sleep apnea was similar to that from diabetes. Research has also found lower death rates among people treated with positive airway pressure therapy, suggesting that the treatment may reduce the risk of death.

WHEN TO SEE A DOCTOR

Snoring. Daytime sleepiness. Morning headaches. These are a few key symptoms of sleep apnea and indications that you should see a doctor. Left untreated, sleep apnea can have severe consequences for your day-to-day well-being and long-term health. But treatments to improve symptoms of sleep apnea can't begin working until you first take the small but crucial step of seeking medical care.

Snoring is a common symptom of obstructive sleep apnea. It's important to let your doctor know that you snore, especially if your snoring is accompanied by daytime sleepiness or other sleep apnea symptoms, such as lack of concentration and irritability.

In addition to nightly snoring and daytime sleepiness, doctors look for a few other key symptoms that can indicate an increased likelihood of obstructive sleep apnea. Gasping or choking during sleep, or your partner noticing that you frequently wake up or stir, is an indication of increased risk for the condition.

In addition to snoring and excessive sleepiness, other reasons to be evaluated for sleep apnea include:

- **Obesity.** Four out of 10 people who are obese have obstructive sleep apnea, and 7 out of 10 people with obstructive sleep apnea are obese.
- **Large neck size.** Your neck size can be an indicator of sleep apnea. Statistically, men with a neck measuring 17 inches or more in circumference and women with a neck of 16 inches or more have an increased likelihood of obstructive sleep apnea. This could be because a larger neck size may be the result of excess fat that contributes to crowding in the throat.
- **Having type 2 diabetes or high blood pressure.** If you have either of these conditions, speak with your doctor about whether you should be evaluated for obstructive sleep apnea, even if you don't have any symptoms.

Keep in mind that you don't need to check off all the boxes for sleep apnea to be at risk. For example, while most people with obstructive sleep apnea are obese, countless slender people are diagnosed with the condition each year.

Snoring

> Thou dost snore distinctly; there's meaning in thy snores.
> —William Shakespeare, "The Tempest"

Snoring can be a nuisance, especially to a bed partner, but it also can signal that something is seriously wrong. Snoring is the most common symptom of obstructive sleep apnea, potentially indicating a serious condition with significant health implications. Loud snoring, or sounds such as gasping or snorting, should raise special concern.

A test done while you sleep — either at home or in a sleep clinic — is the surest way to determine whether your snoring is a sign of a breathing disorder that's disturbing your sleep (see Chapter 5). While snoring is one of the most common symptoms of sleep apnea, just because you snore doesn't mean you have the condition. Snoring that's unrelated to sleep apnea is sometimes called primary or simple snoring.

Snoring is caused by the vibration of soft tissue in your upper airway, and the anatomy of your mouth and throat can make you more likely to snore. A large uvula — the blob of tissue that dangles in front of the opening of your throat — can make you snore. So can a deviated septum, when the bone and cartilage that form the bridge of the nose are displaced to one side, narrowing that airway.

With the exception of pigs and some dog breeds, humans are the only creatures that snore. These guttural nighttime sounds are the collateral result of our ability to carry on a conversation. To accommodate the voice box (larynx), the human airway has a unique anatomy that makes us susceptible to snoring.

COMMON SYMPTOMS OF OBSTRUCTIVE SLEEP APNEA

- Loud snoring.
- Excessive daytime sleepiness.
- A partner notices short halts to your breathing while you sleep.
- Gasping for air during sleep.
- Waking up with a dry mouth.
- Morning headache.
- Difficulty staying asleep.
- Difficulty paying attention during the day.
- Irritability.

In some people, snoring can get extremely loud. According to Guinness World Records, a Swedish man undergoing a sleep study in a hospital in 1993 reached a peak level of 93 decibels, which is louder than a lawn mower.

Many people snore occasionally, perhaps only when they sleep on their back. Alcohol consumption also increases snoring because it relaxes the tissues in the back of your throat. Similarly, some sleep aids, including over-the-counter antihistamines and some prescription medications, can increase snoring.

Snoring tends to be worse during deep sleep, and you may be more likely to snore during catch-up sleep after staying awake for a long time.

Some people are able to quit snoring by cutting back on alcohol, losing weight and avoiding sleeping on their backs.

SNORING

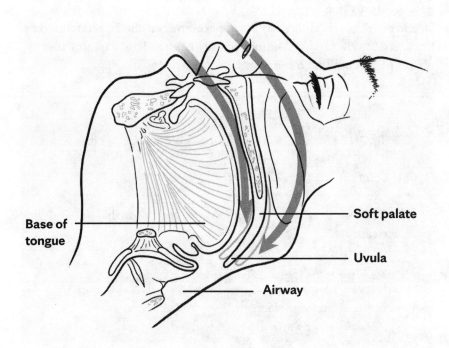

Snoring happens when air flows past relaxed tissues in the throat, causing the tissues, including the uvula, to vibrate and make noise.

For snoring that isn't associated with obstructive sleep apnea, the American Academy of Sleep Medicine and the American Academy of Dental Sleep Medicine recommend that doctors prescribe an oral appliance to treat the snoring. When fitted by a dentist, this device has been shown to reduce snoring and improve sleep and quality of life for snorers as well as for their bed partners. You can read more about it in the next chapter.

Snoring strategies
If you're bothered by snoring, consider taking some of these steps and see if you notice an improvement in how often you snore.
1. **Sleep position.** Sleep on your side, rather than on your back. This can help prevent the tongue and soft palate from collapsing to the back of the throat, which causes snoring.
2. **Weight management.** Maintaining a healthy weight through regular exercise and a balanced diet can prevent fatty tissue from accumulating around the throat, reducing the likelihood of snoring.
3. **Alcohol and sedatives.** Alcohol and sedatives relax the muscles in the throat, increasing the risk of snoring. Limit or avoid these substances, especially close to bedtime.
4. **Hydration.** Drinking plenty of water can help keep the tissues in the throat from becoming sticky, reducing the chances of snoring.
5. **Nasal congestion.** If your nose is congested, use saline nasal sprays or set up a humidifier in the bedroom. Blocked nasal passages can force breathing through the mouth, increasing the risk of snoring. Some people find they can reduce snoring with over-the-counter nasal dilators. These can be special strips that "tent open" the soft parts of the nose, or devices inserted slightly into the nose to prop open the nostrils.
6. **Allergies.** If you have allergies, manage them with allergy medications, such as nonsedating antihistamines or topical nasal steroid sprays. Allergic reactions can lead to nasal congestion and snoring. Avoid nasal or oral decongestants as a regular way to reduce nasal congestion.
7. **Sleep environment.** Sleep with a supportive mattress and pillows that promote proper head and neck alignment.

8. **Throat exercises.** Some people find that throat exercises, such as singing or playing a wind instrument, can help strengthen the muscles in the throat and reduce snoring.
9. **Oral appliances.** Consider using oral appliances designed to keep the airway open and prevent snoring. These devices, discussed in the next chapter, are available over the counter or through a dentist.
10. **Bed elevation.** Raising the head of the bed by a few inches can help keep your airway open and reduce snoring. A few studies show that elevating the head of the bed to a 15- to 30-degree angle can reduce snoring in some people.
11. **Sleep schedule.** Maintain a consistent sleep schedule by going to bed and waking up at the same times each day. This can improve overall sleep quality and reduce snoring.

The effectiveness of these recommendations can vary from person to person. If snoring persists even after you have tried these strategies, or if it becomes a significant concern, see a medical professional or a sleep specialist.

DIAGNOSING SLEEP APNEA

If your doctor believes that you may have obstructive sleep apnea or are at risk for it, the next step will be to work through a methodical process to reach a diagnosis.

This begins with gathering a thorough sleep history, including accounts of snoring, choking, gasping or restlessness during sleep. Your bed partner often can be helpful in providing this information.

Your doctor will want to know if you struggle with excessive daytime sleepiness. You may have a physical exam to evaluate your breathing, heart and nervous system. Your doctor will consider other conditions that are commonly associated with obstructive sleep apnea, including obesity, high blood pressure, congestive heart failure and stroke.

In addition, you may be given a questionnaire to complete (see pages 115 and 117). These screening tools help determine your risk for having obstructive sleep apnea or your degree of sleepiness, which helps your doctor decide if a sleep test is necessary. Because the questionnaires can lead to a relatively high number of false positives or negatives, doctors don't rely on them exclusively to make a diagnosis.

Which test is right for you?
A definitive diagnosis of obstructive sleep apnea can be made only after a sleep test is performed, either at home or in a sleep clinic. Making a diagnosis without a sleep test could result in expensive and burdensome treatment that's unnecessary and ineffective, or in failure to offer treatment to someone who could benefit from it.

There are two types of sleep tests: one that you perform in your own home and the other that's done in a sleep lab or clinic. The test done in the clinic is typically called a sleep study, or polysomnography. The type you complete at home is called a home sleep apnea test.

If your doctor believes you may have moderate or severe obstructive sleep apnea with no complications, then a home sleep apnea test may be appropriate. Home tests are far more convenient than those performed in a lab or clinic, and they may yield sufficient high-quality data about your breathing during sleep to make a diagnosis. This is especially helpful in parts of the country where there isn't a sleep clinic nearby and undergoing a sleep study can be difficult. In some cases, a home sleep apnea test may even be delivered to you by mail after an in-person or telemedicine visit with a doctor.

Sometimes a home sleep test comes back negative or inconclusive, even in people with a high likelihood of having obstructive sleep apnea. In those cases, doctors will generally recommend an overnight sleep study be performed in a sleep clinic.

An overnight sleep test in a clinic is the appropriate choice for people who have other medical conditions that could be related to obstructive sleep apnea. These include certain cardiovascular and respiratory diseases, opioid use, severe insomnia, a sleep-related breathing disorder called hypoventilation and some neuromuscular conditions. A sleep study might also be appropriate if your doctor is concerned that a home sleep apnea test might not be sensitive enough to make a diagnosis. In addition, a sleep study can be helpful in determining how well a person responds to positive airway pressure therapies.

If a sleep study comes back negative despite a high likelihood of obstructive sleep apnea, a second test may be recommended.

Sleep study (polysomnography)

A sleep study, also known as polysomnography, is considered the gold standard for diagnosing obstructive sleep apnea and other sleep disorders. The test is performed overnight as you sleep in an accredited sleep center or hospital (see page 119).

A sleep study consists of many elements. The term *polysomnography* was coined in the 1970s as sleep scientists bundled together several different diagnostic tests to produce a single exam that creates a full portrait of the brain and body during the night. The study provides a wealth of insights into your breathing, heart rate and rhythm, and sleep stages in the course of the night.

A sleep study is most often used to determine if a person has obstructive sleep apnea or other breathing-related disorders, but it also may be used in the diagnosis of other sleep-related conditions, such as narcolepsy, REM sleep behavior disorder, parasomnias that include sleepwalking or talking, and unexplained long-lasting insomnia.

People undergoing a sleep study often worry if they'll be able to sleep in a clinic setting. Nearly everyone does fall asleep during the test. Also, sleep specialists are well aware that a night in a sleep lab — attached to sensors and wires as you try to relax in unfamiliar surroundings — will be quite different from sleeping at home. The test, however, doesn't require a normal night's sleep. Instead, its primary goal is to gather information about your breathing, brain waves, heart rhythms and movements during sleep. Even short periods of sleep — two hours or more — can reveal much to the specialist evaluating your sleep.

What's being monitored?

The components that make up a sleep study focus on several aspects of sleep that may be altered by obstructive sleep apnea. During an overnight stay in a sleep clinic, this is commonly what sleep specialists are monitoring:

- **Brain waves.** They're recorded with a test known as electroencephalography (EEG). Using sensors placed at multiple points on your scalp, this test monitors the electrical activity in the brain that characterizes the different stages of sleep. Breathing disruptions can upset how your body cycles through stages of light, deep and REM sleep. EEG is a key difference between a sleep study performed in a sleep clinic and a home sleep apnea test. Most home sleep apnea tests don't measure brain waves and can't track the stages of sleep and wakefulness precisely.

- **Oxygen levels.** Oxygen in your blood is measured with a pulse oximeter clipped to your finger. A dip in oxygen levels is one of the most harmful effects of obstructive sleep apnea. A pulse oximeter is painless and uses light beamed through your skin to take measurements and gather data.
- **Breathing.** It's measured in multiple ways to reveal different bits of information about apnea episodes. Airflow is measured with pressure sensors at the nostrils. Belts around your chest and stomach measure how much effort is used in breathing, which can help distinguish between obstructive sleep apnea and central sleep apnea.
- **Heart rate and rhythm.** These are tracked with electrocardiography (ECG or EKG) to detect variability or irregular heart rhythm patterns during sleep.
- **Chin muscles.** Activity in the muscles is monitored with a test called electromyography, which uses small sensors to measure changes in muscle tone during different stages of sleep, especially REM.
- **Leg movements.** Sensors placed on your legs measure movement in your lower legs.
- **Eye movement.** Rapid eye movement (REM) is identified and monitored with small sensors attached to the skin near each eye.
- **Body position.** Sensors are placed at specific locations on your body to help determine if your breathing disruptions are related to the way you lie in bed.

A video may be taken while you sleep to help identify unusual movements, behaviors or seizures that may be related to your breathing disorder.

Generally, after just a few hours, a sleep study has gathered enough information to inform a diagnosis. If it appears to the technician overseeing the test that you have obstructive sleep apnea, you may be woken and asked to use a PAP device for the second half of the night. This allows the technician to observe whether the device can prevent apnea episodes and to determine the amount of pressure required to keep your airway open, a process called titration. This is invaluable information for when your treatment begins.

Home sleep apnea tests
While a sleep study is considered the gold standard for sleep tests, home tests are sufficient for many people. A home test is generally best suited for individuals who may have moderate to severe sleep apnea and whose condition is likely to be uncomplicated, meaning that it isn't related to another illness, such as cardiovascular disease.

HAVING A SLEEP STUDY? WHAT TO EXPECT

You'll be provided detailed instructions before you have a sleep study, but here's an example of some of the guidance you may be given prior to your overnight stay and what you can expect:
- Follow your normal daily schedule.
- Don't nap after noon.
- Don't consume caffeine after noon.
- Eat dinner at the usual time.
- Shower or bathe as usual.
- Don't use makeup, lotions, oils, gels, conditioners or other hair products, as these can prevent sensors from sticking to your skin.
- Take any evening medications prior to going to the sleep center.
- If you take a sleep medication, bring this with you to the sleep center.
- Bring something comfortable to sleep in and clothes for the next day.

A doctor will generally determine if you qualify for a home test after gathering your medical history and meeting with you — either in person or via a telemedicine visit — to discuss your symptoms and concerns.

Most people prefer the convenience of sleeping in their own bed during the test instead of going to a sleep center. Numerous studies have demonstrated that home tests can effectively diagnose moderate to severe obstructive sleep apnea in individuals who meet certain criteria after meeting with their doctor. In many cases, insurance will cover a sleep study in a sleep center only after a home test has been performed and is inconclusive or raises new questions.

During a home sleep apnea test, an electronic device is attached to your body while you sleep (see page 120). Home sleep tests are

- At the sleep center, a technician will connect you to the sensors that monitor your body during sleep.
- Sensors that monitor breathing, brain waves, and limb movements are glued to your skin; soft bands that measure breathing are wrapped around your stomach and chest; a device that measures airflow is placed on your face or clipped to your nose; a clip is placed on your finger or ear to measure oxygen levels; a microphone is taped to your neck to record snoring; a video camera may be used to track your sleeping positions.
- If you need to get up during the night for any reason, you'll need to signal to the technician, who can unhook some of the monitoring devices.
- You may be fitted with a positive airway pressure device halfway through the night to see what effect it has. This will allow the technician to determine the pressure needed to keep your airway open.

available in different brands and models, vary from one manufacturer to another and may measure different aspects of sleep. As the hardware and software in the devices advance, manufacturers continue to add new features. The tests are approved by the Food and Drug Administration (FDA) after being determined to be safe and effective.

Most home sleep apnea tests typically monitor the following:
- **Oxygen level.** A device placed on your fingertip or ear measures the percentage of oxygen saturation in your blood. Oxygen saturation is a telling sign of how well you are breathing.
- **Breathing.** Chest movement during breathing is measured via what's called respiratory inductance plethysmography, which uses

AN IMPORTANT BUT INEXACT MEASURE

A diagnosis of obstructive sleep apnea is often characterized as mild, moderate or severe. This determination is generally a result of your apnea-hypopnea index (AHI) score, which is based on the average number of times per hour that your breathing is blocked completely (apnea) or partially (hypopnea) for at least 10 seconds.

Having five or more such events per hour qualifies as mild obstructive sleep apnea; 15 to 30 events per hour is considered moderate; and more than 30 breathing disruptions per hour is called severe.

In reality, apnea episodes aren't evenly distributed throughout the night but tend to be clustered. A diagnosis of obstructive sleep apnea may suggest, for example, that you experience 20 interruptions per hour. However, that doesn't mean you're in fact having an apnea event every three minutes or 20 every hour. The index number represents an average, not a rate. You may go for a long period with no disturbances, then experience several successive awakenings in a relatively short time.

elastic bands to measure the expansion and contraction of your chest.
- **Blood volume.** The amount of blood in tiny arteries is measured with peripheral arterial tonometry (PAT), which can identify breathing disturbances that make the arteries constrict.
- **Movement.** It can be picked up with a test called actigraphy, which helps determine if you're asleep or awake.
- **Nasal pressure.** Some tests monitor nasal pressure by way of a tube fitted with a soft cannula or prongs that is inserted into your nose.

Unlike a sleep study, a home sleep apnea test primarily monitors breathing, not how you cycle through the different sleep stages or

Some home sleep apnea tests provide a different but similar score based on the length of the test, not on how long you were actually asleep.

Many sleep experts believe the AHI measure doesn't adequately capture the severity of sleep apnea for each individual. In fact, the *Journal of Clinical Sleep Medicine* published an article in 2020 titled "When Will We Ditch the AHI?"

One limitation of the AHI is that it can't reliably predict the symptoms and health outcomes of obstructive sleep apnea. In other words, one person told that they have a "severe" case might not feel sleepy during the day and have few apparent health effects, while another might have excessive sleepiness and serious cardiovascular complications.

But while it isn't perfect, the AHI or a similar score is still an important element that your doctor will consider during diagnosis and treatment, in addition to other factors important in determining the severity of your condition. They include your daily vigor, overall health and feeling of well-being.

how long you're asleep. Most home sleep apnea tests, therefore, can't count how many breathing interruptions occurred during total sleep, but instead deliver a number based on breathing interruptions during the test.

Some home tests use pattern recognition to estimate total sleep time and sleep stages. It's not exactly the same as what's measured during a sleep study but can provide additional information that may be helpful. When you've completed the test, you send it to a laboratory where the data is interpreted and reviewed by a sleep medicine specialist.

CENTRAL SLEEP APNEA

We've spent the majority of this chapter discussing the most common form of sleep apnea, obstructive sleep apnea. Central sleep apnea is an uncommon, different form of sleep apnea that also causes frequent interruptions in breathing, resulting in disrupted sleep, reduced blood oxygen levels and increased blood pressure.

Unlike the mechanical blockage of the airway that characterizes obstructive sleep apnea, central sleep apnea is caused by a breakdown in the sensor and signaling system that tells the body to breathe. The result is what doctors call a lack of respiratory effort.

People with central sleep apnea may wake up frequently, have headaches in the morning, be sleepy and fatigued during the day, and suffer from poor concentration. A bed partner might not notice breathing disruptions during sleep because many people with the condition don't snore, a common symptom of obstructive sleep apnea.

Central sleep apnea affects less than 1% of the overall population, though it occurs more frequently among older people. Men are more likely than women to have the condition. It's also possible to have both central and obstructive sleep apnea.

Causes of central sleep apnea

The temporary breathing interruptions associated with central sleep apnea may be triggered by how your body reacts to changes in carbon dioxide in your blood. Just as your blood carries oxygen to feed your cells, it also picks up your cells' waste products, including carbon dioxide, which is expelled through the lungs.

In central sleep apnea, the sensors and signaling system that govern breathing become erratic, swinging from having you breathe too much to having you breathe too little. People with central sleep apnea respond quickly to increases in carbon dioxide in their blood, prompting rapid breathing to eliminate the waste gas through the lungs. When the body senses that carbon dioxide levels have fallen, it slows breathing or halts it altogether, resulting in an apnea event.

There are several types of central sleep apnea. The most common is central sleep apnea with Cheyne-Stokes breathing, which may be associated with heart failure. Heart failure leads to increased fluid around the lungs, which stretches nearby sensors and prompts faster breathing. This upsets the healthy balance of carbon dioxide and oxygen in the blood, prompting breathing to slow or stop. Because you're not breathing, your body eventually rouses you from sleep at least enough to resume breathing again. This begins a new cycle where breathing accelerates, then decelerates, with some periods where breathing stops. These breathing patterns can occur during the day but are more common during sleep.

Central sleep apnea may be triggered by certain medications. People who require opioid pain medication or who abuse opioids are more likely to have central sleep apnea. Certain medical conditions, such as Parkinson's disease and renal failure, also can lead to central sleep apnea. In addition, brain injury or stroke can damage the part of the brain that controls breathing, leading to central sleep apnea.

High-altitude central sleep apnea is another form of the condition that frequently occurs during the first few nights after arrival at a high altitude. It develops before your body can acclimate to the lower oxygen levels in the air. During sleep, your body tries to compensate for the thinner air by breathing a little faster, sending carbon dioxide levels plunging. This prompts the body to stop breathing for a time. Some people with breathing disruptions during sleep are prescribed the medication acetazolamide before traveling to high altitudes to improve their breathing patterns when they arrive.

When no other cause for central sleep apnea can be found, the condition is diagnosed as primary or idiopathic central sleep apnea.

About 1 in 10 people who begin positive airway pressure treatment for obstructive sleep apnea also develop central sleep apnea. When both appear, it's called treatment-emergent central sleep apnea. In most people, the central sleep apnea clears up as positive airway pressure therapy continues.

Diagnosis and treatment of central sleep apnea
An overnight sleep study in a sleep clinic is generally required to diagnose central sleep apnea. While a home sleep apnea test can identify many cases of obstructive sleep apnea, it isn't a preferred way to diagnose central sleep apnea.

First-line treatment for central sleep apnea for individuals with heart failure that isn't too severe is positive airway pressure therapy, often with a continuous positive airway pressure (CPAP) device. If that doesn't work, a special form of positive airway pressure therapy, called adaptive servo-ventilation (ASV), is often the next option. You can read about these devices in the next chapter.

ASV continuously monitors your breathing patterns while you sleep. It's equipped with sensors that can detect normal breathing, shallow breathing or pauses in breathing. Based on this information, the ASV device adjusts the air pressure it delivers. This means that if your breathing becomes irregular or stops, the machine gently provides more air to stimulate breathing. Conversely, when your breathing is stable, it reduces the air pressure, making the therapy both effective and comfortable. This dynamic adjustment helps maintain a consistent breathing pattern throughout the night, leading to better sleep quality and overall health.

Despite several studies, it isn't clear whether positive airway pressure treatment improves the overall survival rate for heart failure. But it is clear the treatment can improve some symptoms associated with sleep apnea that can interfere with quality of life, including daytime sleepiness and fatigue.

Among individuals with more severe heart disease, ASV might not be a suitable treatment for central sleep apnea. Some people benefit instead from treatment with an implant that stimulates the phrenic nerve, which governs the diaphragm and the rhythms of breathing. This relatively new treatment uses a device the size of a pacemaker and has been shown to improve symptoms of central sleep apnea in people with heart failure, regardless of severity. The FDA approved a device called remedē System for this treatment in 2017.

Supplemental oxygen and medications, including hypnotics such as zolpidem, can increase sleep and reduce the number of apnea episodes in some people. However, no medications are approved specifically to treat central sleep apnea.

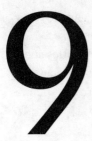

Treating sleep apnea

"It's just part of me." Lauren can say that now, but when she first tried using a breathing device to treat her sleep apnea, things didn't go too well. The mask that fit over her mouth and nose was a big part of the problem, leaving marks on her face in the morning. The pressure from the continuous positive away pressure (CPAP) machine also felt uncomfortable.

But during doctor visits for other health conditions, including COVID-19, she learned that her oxygen saturation was dipping low. It was clear that she needed to do something to improve her obstructive sleep apnea.

Working with her doctor, she switched to a different device, known as a bilevel positive airway pressure (BPAP) device, which increases pressure during inhalation, then ratchets the pressure down during exhalation. The device suited her breathing much better.

Just as important, she didn't use a full mask this time. Instead, she switched to a small, soft nasal pillow that fits beneath her nose and has cushions that fit into her nostrils. It's secured on her head with straps and attached to tubes connected to her bilevel positive airway pressure device. She adjusts the pressure until it's right, then hardly knows it's there.

A smartphone app that's connected to her device also allows Lauren to check her score every morning. Most mornings, it tells her she had no breathing disruptions during the night.

Lauren, who works in higher education, can feel the difference the treatment makes.

"Cognitively, I am able to focus a little more and my brain is a little clearer," she said. "It was a big shift. I felt I was waking up feeling more refreshed from sleep."

Lauren uses a wheelchair, and she said that has shown her how medical devices can transform your life for the better.

"I am a big believer that medical devices are assistive for quality of health and quality of life," she said. "I view the wheelchair as doing that for me, and I believe the BPAP does the same thing."

The lesson for everyone, she said, is that it sometimes it takes trial and error to get the maximum benefit from the device and the treatment.

"You should speak up and advocate for what you need," said Lauren. "It is not one-size-fits-all. You have to experiment to see what works for you."

Obstructive sleep apnea is a serious condition, but it's also highly treatable. Taking care of your sleep apnea is an important step toward improving not only your sleep but your overall health and your quality of life as well. Concentration, productivity at work and even personal relationships can all benefit with treatment.

If your sleep apnea makes you sleepy during the day, alertness and vigor can make a welcome return. And if your sleep apnea is placing you at risk of other serious health conditions, treatment can reduce those risks. Notably, treating sleep apnea can reduce high blood pressure, similar to what you can expect from taking blood pressure medication.

Presently, treatment is recommended for anyone with 15 or more breathing disruptions per hour, or for anyone who has at least 5 breathing disruptions per hour plus other symptoms. These can include daytime sleepiness, problems concentrating, irritability, or co-existing conditions such as low blood pressure, stroke or heart disease.

If you've been diagnosed with sleep apnea but are experiencing few symptoms, you may wonder if treatment is even necessary. Think about it like you would a diagnosis of high cholesterol or high blood pressure. Even though you may not have any symptoms, treating the condition is critical because it can prevent cardiovascular disease and help you live longer and better.

There are several treatment options for obstructive sleep apnea. It's important to discuss them with your doctor to find the one best suited for you. These options include lifestyle changes and weight loss. Medications typically aren't part of sleep apnea treatment, though they can play an indirect role in overall treatment by helping some people fall asleep at night or stay awake during the day.

The most commonly used and predictably effective therapy for obstructive sleep apnea is positive airway pressure (PAP). PAP treatment is often referred to as CPAP, a specific form of PAP therapy known as continuous positive airway pressure. When used regularly, positive airway pressure treatment can reduce or end the regular breathing disruptions that occur during your sleep. It also brings other health benefits.

Positive airway pressure devices provide successful results for a large majority of people who try them. However, a significant number of people who start the treatment find it difficult to get used to and to continue for the long term. Understand that finding the right device and equipment can take patience and some trial and error, but it's important to stick with it.

In the remainder of this chapter, we'll discuss how you can improve your chances of reaping the benefits of sleep apnea treatment. We'll also review other treatment options and approaches that have been shown to improve obstructive sleep apnea.

LIFESTYLE CHANGES

If your sleep apnea is considered mild, your doctor may recommend only lifestyle changes, such as losing weight or quitting smoking.

Perhaps you need to change the position in which you sleep. If you have nasal allergies, treatment for your allergies may improve your sleep apnea.

Lifestyle changes are important, regardless of the severity of your condition. When combined with other forms of treatment, a healthy change in habits, especially a reduction in weight, can help improve your symptoms.

Weight loss

Obesity is a chronic disease that can be influenced by lifestyle, and it's also a well-known risk factor for obstructive sleep apnea. Losing weight can be an effective way to reduce nighttime breathing problems.

Even modest weight loss can help. In one study, weight loss of 10% led to a 26% decrease in the average number of sleep disturbances. Other research shows that more than half of people with mild sleep apnea who lose more than 20 pounds may resolve their symptoms altogether. Even if losing weight doesn't relieve all your apnea disturbances, it can provide other health benefits.

Bariatric surgery, which reduces the size of the stomach to promote weight loss, can reduce the number of apnea episodes and, in a few cases, may allow people to stop using their breathing devices. Most people who require a breathing device before bariatric surgery, however, need to continue using it after the surgery and subsequent weight loss.

Researchers are investigating whether the weight-loss medication semaglutide (Ozempic, Rybelsus, Wegovy) might also be effective for reducing obstructive sleep apnea. Semaglutide medications, which are revolutionizing the treatment of obesity, work by stimulating insulin secretion, decreasing appetite and slowing the emptying of the stomach. Many studies are underway to determine how semaglutide might affect other conditions related to obesity, including breathing disruptions during sleep.

Exercise can reduce obstructive sleep apnea symptoms, even apart from its impact on weight. Studies have shown that full-body aerobic exercise produced moderate improvement of obstructive sleep apnea even when the participants didn't lose weight.

Anyone who's excessively overweight and has obstructive sleep apnea will likely benefit from losing weight. For some people with mild obstructive sleep apnea, losing weight might be enough to eliminate the problem altogether.

Other strategies
In addition to weight loss, other lifestyle changes that may help improve sleep apnea include:
- **Exercise.** Engaging in regular physical activity can strengthen your heart and lungs, improve your energy levels and potentially ease apnea symptoms.
- **A healthy diet.** Eating healthy can support weight management and is important to overall health. Eat a balanced diet rich in fruits, vegetables, whole grains and lean proteins.
- **Changing sleep positions.** Experiment with different sleeping positions. Sleeping on your side, rather than on your back, can reduce the likelihood of airway obstruction.
- **Avoiding alcohol and sedatives.** They can relax the muscles in your throat, increasing the risk of airway collapse during sleep.
- **Stopping smoking.** If you smoke, try to quit. Smoking can increase inflammation and fluid retention in the upper airway, worsening obstructive sleep apnea symptoms.
- **Maintaining a sleep schedule.** Establish a consistent sleep routine — going to bed and waking up at the same time — to improve the quality of your sleep. For additional tips on improving sleep quality, see Chapter 4.

Lifestyle changes are generally most beneficial when combined with other treatments for sleep apnea, such as positive airway pressure therapy.

UNDERSTANDING POSITIVE AIRWAY PRESSURE

For more than four decades, positive airway pressure has proven to be a highly effective treatment for obstructive sleep apnea. And over all these years, manufacturers have been improving the equipment associated with this therapy, making it quieter, easier to use and more comfortable.

PAP works by providing the air you breathe through your nose or mouth at a higher pressure, which physically props open the throat to prevent it from closing and cutting off the flow of air. The pressure delivered by PAP devices is very low, though noticeable. A CPAP

POSITIVE AIRWAY PRESSURE TREATMENT

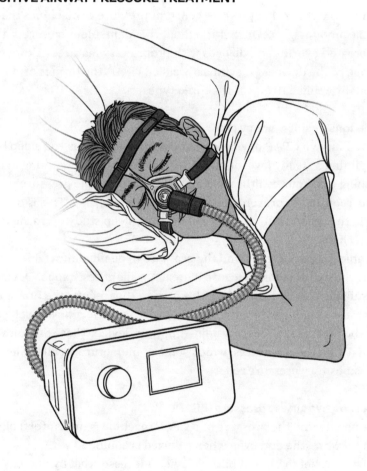

A positive airway pressure (PAP) device delivers steady air pressure to help you breathe while you sleep. Components include the PAP machine, a mask and a hose that connects the machine to the mask.

Treating sleep apnea 211

machine, for example, is typically set to 9 cm H2O, or about 0.13 pounds of force per square inch. For comparison, the pressure in a car tire is typically about 32 pounds, or about 250 times greater than this.

For many people, positive airway pressure treatment often reduces the number of apnea episodes to fewer than five per hour. Other benefits of this treatment, according to research, include reductions in sleepiness, car crashes and high blood pressure. The treatment can also lead to improved quality of life.

There are three primary types of positive airway pressure devices, ranging from those that produce constant pressure to machines that vary the amount of pressure throughout the night. Manufacturers also have created hybrids and devices with proprietary features. Although only one of the devices is technically called CPAP, the term is often informally applied to any of the three types.

Continuous positive airway pressure (CPAP)
The well-known CPAP device keeps your airway open as you sleep by maintaining a steady level of pressure, whether you're breathing in or breathing out. Your healthcare team will determine the pressure setting required to prevent your airway from collapsing. This is often done in the second half of the night during a sleep study performed in a sleep clinic.

Some people say they find the pressure to be uncomfortable during the exhale phase because it creates a slight resistance. Devices are available that address this with a feature that relaxes the pressure slightly each time you breathe out. Typically, you select how much you want the pressure reduced by adjusting your device. These are known as exhalation relief features, which some manufacturers call C-Flex or EPR (expository pressure relief).

Bilevel positive airway pressure (BPAP)
Some people find the pressure of a CPAP machine is uncomfortable when they breathe out, even when a device is equipped with an exhalation relief feature. A bilevel device addresses that by decreasing the air pressure significantly after each breath, reducing resistance to exhalation. After the device is set to the pressure you need to keep your airway open while breathing in, a second, lower level is set for

when you breathe out. This setting is typically lower than that used in devices with exhalation relief. The device then toggles between these two preset levels as you breathe through the night.

Automatic positive airway pressure (APAP)

CPAP and bilevel devices are set at constant pressure levels based on an assessment of what it takes to keep your airway open. In reality, the required level of pressure changes through the night, varying as you shift position and pass through different stages of sleep. Automatic positive airway pressure devices use electronics to sense when your breathing becomes disrupted and raise the pressure to meet what is needed at that moment to keep your airway open.

COMPARING DEVICES

In recent years, APAP has become the most commonly used type of positive airway pressure device. In one analysis, 50% of the people getting treatment used APAP, 41% used CPAP, and the remaining 9% used bilevel or another type.

Changes in how sleep tests are performed are likely the reason that APAP use has increased. Sleep studies done in a clinic can determine the minimum amount of air pressure required to keep the airway open, a number needed before CPAP treatment can begin. This can't be done with a home sleep apnea test. Someone diagnosed with obstructive sleep apnea after a home sleep test will likely be prescribed an APAP machine, which is equipped to find the pressure needed to keep your airway open on its own. The large increase in the use of home sleep apnea tests has subsequently spurred increased use of APAP.

While some people prefer the variability of APAP and find it more comfortable, others say changes in air pressure throughout the night interrupt their sleep. For these individuals, CPAP may be the better option. Success rates involving positive airway pressure treatment don't vary much according to the type of device used, though some studies have found that people might use an APAP device a bit longer each night.

Some studies indicate that CPAP is more effective than APAP at reducing the risk of certain serious health conditions, including high blood pressure. This isn't yet well understood, but researchers have explored whether changes in pressure throughout the night with APAP devices might disturb sleep with microarousals, reducing the benefit of the treatment. For people who aren't finding success with APAP, switching to CPAP can sometimes improve their results.

YOUR EQUIPMENT: CLEANING AND TRAVELING

Positive airway pressure devices require maintenance and supplies, which can include mask wipes and brushes for cleaning the tubing. Regular cleaning is necessary to prevent bacteria from growing inside the equipment. Also, because the mask touches your face or nose all night, manufacturers recommend that it be washed with soap and water every morning. Hoses are typically washed with soap and water once or twice a week. The humidifier tank that's now standard on many devices can usually be placed in the top rack of the dishwasher weekly.

When traveling, some people rent or buy a portable positive airway pressure device rather than use their home machine. Travel devices are sometimes made smaller by eliminating the humidifier feature or using an alternative type of humidifier that doesn't require a tank. Many people, however, find they aren't as effective as the heated humidifier on their home machine and prefer to travel with their day-to-day device.

Regular PAP machines often fit into a pack that resembles a briefcase for a laptop computer, and they can be carried aboard an airplane and stowed under the seat in front of you or in the overhead bin. Because the machine is classified as an assistive device, the Federal Aviation Administration prohibits airlines from counting your PAP machine in its case as an additional piece of carry-on luggage.

Your doctor will work with you to help determine which type of device to begin with and may make a recommendation about which model to use. Staff at a reliable medical equipment store also have expertise in the devices. Ultimately, the most important factor for you to consider when choosing a device is which one you are most comfortable using.

STICKING WITH TREATMENT

Research and experience convincingly show that positive airway pressure is a highly successful treatment that can improve your health and make you feel better. The vast majority of people who start the treatment keep using it. About three-quarters of the people who begin treatment with positive airway pressure are still using it at least four hours or more per night on most nights three months later. (We recommend you use the device all night, every night.)

Over the years, there have been many improvements in the devices, masks and hoses, addressing many earlier issues with the treatment. The machines are much quieter — similar to the sound of a whisper — than earlier models. The masks are more comfortable. The addition of adjustable humidity systems prevents your nose and mouth from drying out. And heated tubing keeps the moisture in humid air from forming into annoying droplets.

Yet while some people can't sleep without their device, others can't sleep with it. Over the long haul, the number of people who continue to use positive airway pressure treatment declines. Studies suggest that about one-third of the people who start the treatment eventually discontinue it. People with the most severe symptoms, including sleepiness and low blood oxygen levels, are those most likely to stay the course.

Positive airway pressure treatment is a therapy, not a cure. In most cases it must be continued for life to keep providing benefits. There may be times when you need to remind yourself that the treatment is vital to your overall health and daily wellness.

There are steps you can take to help ensure that you stick with the treatment. We'll provide some concrete tips to help you find a comfortable, well-fitted mask and other practical ways to improve your treatment experience.

The all-important mask

Most people receiving treatment for sleep apnea use a PAP device. Finding the right mask is one of the most important aspects of treatment — and also the most difficult. Know that it may take some trial and error before you find the mask that works best for you.

MEDICARE AND INSURANCE COVERAGE

Private insurance or Medicare typically covers at least part of the cost of sleep apnea devices and their supplies. If you have private insurance, contact your insurer to learn about your coverage.

Medicare has some coverage requirements. If you're diagnosed with obstructive sleep apnea and are prescribed treatment with positive airway pressure, Medicare may cover a three-month trial period, then will continue to cover some of the cost if you meet certain conditions. These conditions, according to rules currently in effect, include seeing your doctor, who must document that the treatment is helping you.

Original Medicare will pay 80% of the cost of the rental of a positive airway pressure device and its supplies once you've met the Part B deductible. Medicare will pay the rental for 13 months if you continue to regularly use the treatment, and at the end of that rental period you will own the machine.

Medicare covers CPAP, BPAP, APAP and oral appliances if prescribed by your doctor, but it will only cover one treatment option at a time. It's also important that both your doctor and the equipment supplier accept Medicare. While the vast majority do, Medicare advises you to check first to make certain you're not responsible for the entire cost.

Many people are anxious about sleeping with a mask at night. You've likely seen pictures of PAP machines showing large face masks that look like what a fighter pilot might wear. The prospect of wearing such a device each night may have you nervous and concerned. Don't be! A wide array of mask styles and models is now available, and many of them have a relatively low profile and attach to your nose, not your mouth.

In fact, there are so many masks on the market — more than 200 — that choosing one can be a daunting challenge. Some masks fit over the mouth and nose (oronasal). Some are placed over just the nose (nasal). And others fit beneath the nose and rest in the nostrils (nasal pillow). Straps that go with these masks can vary from a single band around the back of the head to a three-strap harness that keeps the mask secure.

Many sleep experts recommend starting with a nasal mask. Nasal masks can require lower levels of pressure to keep the airway open, which many people find more comfortable. Some studies suggest that people who use a nasal mask are more likely to use their device the entire night than those who use other types. Research also suggests that nasal masks lead to fewer apnea events during sleep, which can be seen in lower AHI scores.

Many people find the nasal pillow style works best for them and is the least restrictive and obtrusive.

If you breathe through your mouth, you may be concerned that a nasal mask won't work for you. Indeed, when you snore, you're most likely breathing through your mouth. However, positive airway pressure through the nose keeps the airway open, averting snoring. It seals the soft palate in the back of the mouth against the base of the tongue, preventing mouth breathing in most people. Plus, many people who believe they're breathing through their mouth might in fact be breathing through their nose.

In those cases where a person is a mouth breather but still wants to use a nasal mask, a chin strap or special tape can be used to keep the mouth closed. Though it might sound like an extreme remedy, many people find it to be comfortable and effective. For some people who breathe through their mouth, the oronasal mask is the best option.

When getting your PAP equipment, it's important to visit a reputable dealer with expertise in fitting masks. If you aren't satisfied with the quality of the service, try another retail store if your insurance allows it.

Also, make sure to check the return policy on the mask you're considering. Some manufacturers allow a 30-day trial and will refund your money if the mask doesn't work well. About one-third of people who start treatment switch out their mask within three months.

Proper fit is crucial because the mask must be sealed to your face. Even small leaks can interfere with the effectiveness of the treatment and cause irritation at the site of the leak. To help with mask discomfort, try petroleum-free skin moisturizers, nasal saline sprays, oral rinses for dry mouth or liners for the mask.

Many people switch masks several times. Finding the right mask isn't unlike finding a comfortable exercise shoe. The fit might feel right in the store, but it takes some use at home to determine if it's the right one for you.

FINDING A MASK WITH YOUR PHONE

You use your cellphone for a lot of things, but you probably didn't expect that it could help you find the right mask for your PAP machine.

Many cellphones are equipped with facial recognition software that scans and measures your face. With the use of a downloadable app, those capabilities can be used to compare the dimensions and unique contours of your face with a database of mask sizes and measurements.

Manufacturers have produced apps for their lines of products, and independent developers offer apps that can compare your face against multiple mask brands and even include customer reviews.

MASK STYLES

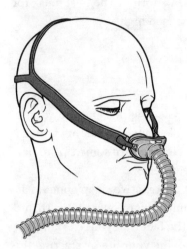

A nasal pillow mask fits at the nostrils.

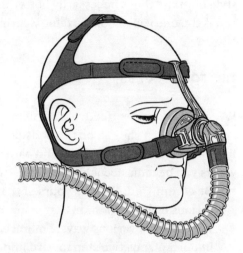

A nasal mask covers the nose.

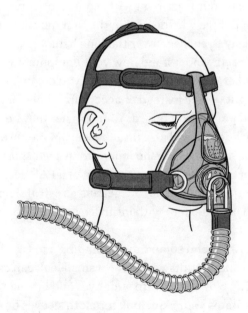

A full-face (oronasal) mask covers the nose and mouth.

Once you find the right mask style and fit, stick with it. There is no style or brand that's necessarily better than another. The best mask for you is the one you're comfortable wearing each night.

TIPS FOR SUCCESS

PAP devices are an effective treatment for sleep apnea, but they don't do much good if they sit on the bedside table unused. Sleeping with a PAP machine often takes time and patience. Here are some tips to help you as you become accustomed to the treatment:

- **Be committed.** Remind yourself that obstructive sleep apnea is a serious health condition that compromises your overall health and well-being in various ways. Embrace the fact that you're taking an important, positive step toward improving your life by starting this treatment and sticking with it.
- **Set yourself up for success.** It's important to get off to a good start. Approach your treatment with a positive attitude. Research suggests that people who do well in the first month or two are the ones most likely to succeed over the long haul.
- **Educate yourself.** Understand how your equipment works and become familiar with its features before you begin. Make an effort to find the right device instead of accepting whatever you're given.
- **Get your bed partner on board.** Your partner may be anxious about how the device will affect their sleep. Make sure they know how quiet the machines are (no louder than a whisper). In fact, many bed partners prefer the quiet hum of a PAP device to the loud snoring that kept them from getting a restful sleep. PAP devices need not interfere with intimacy and sex. They're worn only during sleep.
- **Seek a good fit.** Spend some time on finding a mask you're comfortable with and that fits well. Even a small leak can cause problems, including blowing air into your eyes and drying them out. If your mask irritates your skin, look for cloth sleeves or small pads that cushion the mask against your skin.
- **Get comfortable with the mask.** Before you need to use it, take some simple steps to get used to the mask. During the day, put it

on with the machine off. Then turn on the machine for a bit to experience the pressure sensation. Knowing what to expect may lessen your anxiety when it's time to sleep.
- **Consider using the "ramp" feature.** This setting, which is common on most devices, is used when you're first going to sleep. It starts at a low pressure, then gradually ramps it up to acclimate you as you fall asleep.
- **Adjust the humidity with the seasons.** Experiment with the humidity feature to make the treatment more comfortable and to reduce the throat dryness and nasal dryness and congestion that can be side effects of PAP therapy. The humidity feature also helps prevent your eyes from drying.
- **Don't let your mask come off during the night.** If you repeatedly find your mask is off when you wake up in the morning, try the alarm feature on your device, if it has one. This will wake you if the mask comes off or you unconsciously take it off. This will often train you to stop taking the mask off during sleep.
- **Leave the mask on when you use the bathroom.** Rather than taking off the mask when you get out of bed during the night, just disconnect the hose. This will make it easier and quicker to get back into bed and reduce the likelihood that you'll just leave the mask off for the rest of the night.
- **Give it time.** This is new, and there's a learning curve. Your equipment might take some getting used to. Don't give up.
- **Don't expect immediate results.** Some symptoms of obstructive sleep apnea, such as snoring or gasping for air, should disappear quickly. Others, such as daytime sleepiness and mental fogginess, might linger for a few weeks or longer.
- **Be a problem solver.** Problems are sure to crop up. Don't be overwhelmed. Instead, concentrate on handling just one matter at a time. When you solve that, you can work on the next.
- **Get help.** If you're struggling with treatment for your sleep apnea or having difficulty sleeping, discuss it with your doctor. Your doctor or members of the medical staff may be able to offer solutions to your problems. In addition, in certain situations, a doctor may prescribe sleep medication for a short time as you get used to sleeping with a PAP device.

ORAL APPLIANCES

Another treatment for obstructive sleep apnea uses a specially fitted mouthpiece that helps keep your airway open by shifting your jaw slightly forward. Oral appliances are most often recommended for people with mild obstructive sleep apnea who either don't want to use positive airway pressure treatment or can't use it. In some cases, an oral appliance can be effective for people with moderate or even severe obstructive sleep apnea.

An oral appliance isn't as successful at lowering the number of apnea episodes during the night as positive airway pressure is. But among those individuals who are more likely to use an oral appliance than a PAP device, the therapy can be effective.

If your doctor believes an oral appliance may be appropriate for you, you'll be referred to a dentist who will oversee the fit and the

ORAL APPLIANCE

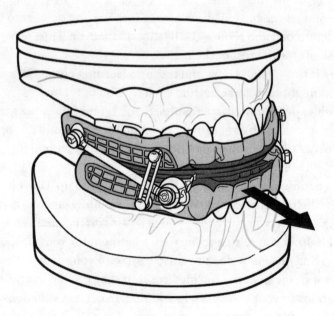

Oral appliances open your airway by pulling your jaw forward.

manufacture of your device. A dentist also can do an overall evaluation of your mouth to determine if you're a good candidate for the device.

Being an appropriate candidate includes having enough healthy teeth — preferably at least several upper and lower teeth on both sides of the mouth — to keep the appliance in place as you sleep. Your jaw must also be able to move forward far enough for the device to work effectively. If you meet the criteria for an oral device, images of your teeth and jaw will be converted into a digital impression that's used to mold the device.

Once you have the appliance, you'll be instructed on how to adjust it regularly, gradually getting it to the point where it's moving your jaw forward the desired amount. Some people are given a second device to wear for a short time early in the morning to help realign the jaw after wearing the appliance all night.

Like any treatment, oral appliances can have unwanted side effects. They can cause jaw discomfort, result in too much salivation or lead to a dry mouth. Over time, the device can affect the position of your teeth, so regular follow-up care with your dentist is required.

People who do adapt to the use of an oral appliance like it for its simplicity, including the fact that it's easy to travel with.

However, because manufacturing a custom oral appliance to treat sleep apnea can be complex, these devices are expensive. They can easily cost more than twice the price of a PAP machine. These costs are typically covered by Medicare or private insurance as a medical expense, not as a dental expense.

SURGERY

In cases where positive airway pressure treatment or an oral appliance may not be appropriate, other options may be considered, including surgery. There are several types of surgery that have been used to treat obstructive sleep apnea with varying degrees of success.

Bariatric surgery

Bariatric surgery isn't a primary therapy for obstructive sleep apnea, but it can play a role in improving or potentially curing the condition in people who are excessively overweight. Being overweight can contribute to obstructive sleep apnea by increasing fatty tissue around the upper airway, making it more susceptible to collapse during sleep.

In bariatric surgery, the stomach is made smaller, limiting food intake. This typically results in weight loss, reducing the amount of fatty tissue around the upper airway and making the airway less prone to collapse.

Bariatric surgery can also lead to improvement of other health conditions associated with both obesity and obstructive sleep apnea, including high blood pressure, diabetes and cardiovascular disease.

In some cases, particularly when obstructive sleep apnea is directly linked to obesity, significant weight loss following bariatric surgery can bring an end to sleep apnea altogether. However, not all people who undergo bariatric surgery experience a complete cure of obstructive sleep apnea, and the degree of improvement can vary. Even after surgery, many people may still require positive airway pressure therapy or other treatments for obstructive sleep apnea. Whether you need ongoing treatment is often determined by a sleep study done sometime after the bariatric surgery. Long-term monitoring of your breathing is crucial, as weight gain or other factors could lead to the return of obstructive sleep apnea.

The interplay between weight loss, sleep apnea and overall health is complex and requires a comprehensive, individualized approach. People who've undergone bariatric surgery and believe their obstructive sleep apnea is cured should talk to their doctor about having a follow-up sleep study to confirm this.

Soft tissue surgery

This type of surgery includes a procedure called uvulopalatopharyngoplasty (UPPP). It removes some of the soft, flexible structures at the back of the throat that can collapse during sleep, closing off the airway and causing snoring or obstructive breathing. A surgeon may also remove the tonsils and adenoids and trim away other soft tissues, including all or part of the uvula that hangs down at the opening to the throat.

UPPP is the most commonly performed surgery for obstructive sleep apnea, but the procedure isn't always successful. Studies indicate its success rate varies from about 40% to 60%, depending on how carefully patients were selected for the procedure and how success was defined. Some people who find the procedure successful at first see the improvements fade and obstructive sleep apnea return. In earlier versions of this procedure, 44% of people who underwent it experienced an increase in the number of apnea events, the opposite of the intended effect. Changes to the procedure have allowed surgeons to individualize the approach to each person's anatomy, improving success rates.

Complications from this surgery can include bleeding and pain. Recovery can be painful and take several months.

Maxillomandibular advancement surgery
This surgery repositions the upper and lower bones of the jaw to increase the size of the airway. The procedure is sometimes called double jaw surgery. It also alters some muscles and soft tissues to further expand the airway.

Maxillomandibular advancement surgery has been shown to reduce sleep apnea events by an average of about 80%. In half of people with moderate to severe obstructive sleep apnea who have this procedure, the average number of apnea events is reduced to the normal range of five or fewer per hour.

The surgery is generally performed on people who can't use or tolerate positive airway pressure therapy. It can also benefit people with very short lower jaws, a condition known as retrognathia. In moving the jaw permanently forward, the surgery can alter a person's appearance, and many people feel their appearance is improved.

The surgery has also proven successful for people whose obstructive sleep apnea is caused by excess soft tissue or obesity. It takes several hours to complete the procedure, which moves the jaw forward about 0.3 inch. A brief hospital stay is required, and recovery at home takes about six weeks, with the full results apparent in 9 to 12 months.

Complications can include some numbness in the chin caused by trauma to nerves in the jaw during the procedure.

Upper airway stimulation
This form of surgery involves implantation of an electronic device that stimulates the nerves that keep your airway open. The device is marketed as Inspire.

The genioglossus muscle is responsible for moving your tongue as you chew, swallow and speak, and it also plays a big role in whether your airway remains open during sleep. The muscle receives its signals from the hypoglossal nerve, which originates in the brain and runs under the tongue.

Several years ago, the Food and Drug Administration (FDA) approved Inspire, a device that signals the hypoglossal nerve to stimulate the genioglossus muscle under certain conditions, stiffening the tongue and moving it forward. The signal is generated by a small module implanted beneath the collarbone, about the size of a heart pacemaker, which is sometimes implanted in a similar location.

The Inspire module is usually implanted during an outpatient procedure and you go home shortly afterward. It has a respiratory sensor attached to a wire tunneled under the skin to an area on the chest, where it can detect breathing. A stimulation lead is also tunneled up to meet the hypoglossal nerve. Because the device and its two leads are

NERVE STIMULATION

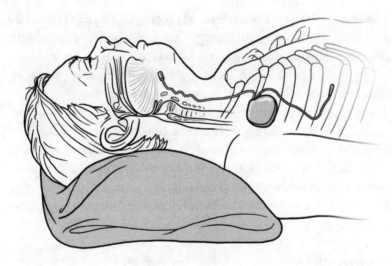

A small module is implanted near the collarbone. One attachment monitors breathing. The other is equipped with a small stimulator that controls tongue movement to help keep the airway open.

completely under the skin, it can be switched on and off only with a remote control.

Before you can have this procedure, doctors must first make sure you're a good candidate. This is done by examining your upper airway while under anesthesia in a procedure called an endoscopy. Additionally, there's a weight cutoff. Individuals with a body mass index above 40 are excluded from the surgery because it's likely to be ineffective.

A well-known study found that approximately two-thirds of the people using Inspire experienced a reduction in breathing disruptions by half or more. On average, the stimulator reduced the number of breathing disruptions from 29 to 9 when measured after one year.

The device is approved by the FDA only for individuals who have moderate to severe obstructive sleep apnea and have tried using a PAP device but are unable to use or tolerate it.

Deviated septum surgery
Surgery to repair a deviated septum or other problems in the nose isn't a direct treatment for obstructive sleep apnea, but it can sometimes help people succeed with other forms of therapy. A deviated septum can increase resistance in the nasal airway and lead to mouth breathing, which can prompt the airway to collapse. Surgery to address these issues may reduce some symptoms of obstructive sleep apnea or make it easier for you to use PAP devices.

POSITIONAL THERAPY

Sleeping on your back (supine position) invites gravity to pull at the soft tissues of your airway, narrowing or closing the airway and interrupting your breathing. Most people with obstructive sleep apnea have at least twice as many breathing disruptions while sleeping on their backs versus on their sides or front.

Positional therapy is a low-risk treatment that prevents you from sleeping on your back. It helps some people reduce the number of times they wake during the night due to breathing disruptions. Studies have shown that positional therapy is effective at reducing apnea episodes and alleviating daytime sleepiness.

While positive airway pressure therapy is generally more effective at improving apnea symptoms, people are often more accepting of positional therapy. Some people use their PAP devices only part of the night (although all night is recommended and preferable); therefore, using both treatments can be beneficial for some individuals.

According to some studies, positional therapy can be as effective as positive airway pressure treatment for people who almost exclusively have apnea episodes while sleeping on their backs, known as positional obstructive sleep apnea. A sleep study in a clinic or a home sleep apnea test can help assess how your sleeping position affects your breathing.

Positional therapy relies on devices that range from high-tech to decidedly low-tech. The simplest is a time-proven trick used to reduce snoring: Attach a tennis ball to the back of what you wear to bed, and the discomfort of the lump beneath you will keep you from rolling onto your back during sleep.

The same lump-in-your-back concept is employed by devices that have inflatable bags attached to a harness that's worn like a backpack. These are available online, often marketed as remedies for snoring. One version, called Zzoma, is available by prescription only. It's worn around the chest and has a soft protrusion on the back.

While many people embrace this approach for its simplicity, some find the lump to be annoying and disruptive to their sleep. Many people quit using it.

Electronic devices for positional therapy are becoming increasingly sophisticated, raising hope they could become even more effective for many people. The devices may rely on thermometers, accelerometers and microchips to monitor when you're sleeping on your back, then vibrate to persuade you to change position. Some people are more likely to use electronic devices than they are a tennis ball on their back.

One electronic device for positional therapy, called NightBalance, is designed to train you to sleep on your side, not on your back. Available only by prescription, it uses a small device that slips into a belt that you wear around your chest to monitor your sleeping position. It begins vibrating if you roll onto your back, and the vibrations gradually increase until they prompt you to change positions, without waking you.

WHAT ABOUT CANNABIS? CAN IT TREAT OBSTRUCTIVE SLEEP APNEA?

As cannabis has become legalized across the United States, some people have come to use it to treat obstructive sleep apnea. However, there's no evidence that cannabis is a safe and effective treatment, and it can produce many potentially negative side effects.

In 2017, the state of Minnesota listed obstructive sleep apnea as one of the conditions that qualify for treatment with medical cannabis. The American Academy of Sleep Medicine responded with a statement that cannabis "should not be used for the treatment of obstructive sleep apnea" and asked that the condition be taken off the list. The organization said there was insufficient evidence that cannabis was safe and effective, and its delivery methods were unreliable.

Some studies of a synthetic cannabis product called dronabinol have shown mixed results, as well as some troubling side effects. Dronabinol is approved by the FDA for treating nausea and vomiting in people undergoing chemotherapy and in treating weight loss in people with acquired immunodeficiency syndrome (AIDS). The compound also affects the nerves that stimulate the tongue, which can play a role in obstructive sleep apnea. Researchers warn that early test results aren't sufficient to show that synthetic cannabis is a safe or effective treatment for obstructive sleep apnea.

There are several potential adverse effects from using cannabis to treat obstructive sleep apnea. Cannabis taken at night can cause sleepiness during the day. Cannabis use is also associated with a higher risk of having an automobile crash. In addition, cannabis and dronabinol are associated with increased appetite and eating, encouraging weight gain, which can increase the symptoms of obstructive sleep apnea.

10

Narcolepsy and idiopathic insomnia

Even in middle school, Daiton felt tired all the time, taking naps whenever she could. Through high school, she drank cup after cup of coffee, though it did little to help her stay awake. When she started college, she would head back to her room to nap between classes.

For Daiton, sleepiness was constant and overpowering. She described it to others as being like a weighted blanket holding her down or a heavy stone on her chest. Although Daiton had felt this way for nearly as long as she could remember, she eventually realized that something was wrong. "That's when I said, 'This is not normal, I have to do something.'" At age 18, she made an appointment with a sleep specialist.

To understand what was making Daiton so sleepy, the specialist performed two different kinds of sleep tests. One was an overnight sleep study (polysomnography), which measures sleep stages and breathing patterns. The other was a daytime test, called a multiple sleep latency test, that measures how long it takes to fall asleep. Her physician also gathered a detailed sleep history and looked for other causes for her sleepiness.

Daiton was diagnosed with idiopathic hypersomnia, a condition without a known cause that produces excessive, even debilitating sleepiness. The diagnosis ended years of questions and self-doubt. "It was vindicating," she said. "I am not crazy, and I am not lazy."

Daiton was started on medication to help her feel awake and alert during the day. "It helped a little, but it didn't work great," she said. Her doctor then switched her to a commonly prescribed medication that promotes wakefulness, which quickly and dramatically reduced her daytime sleepiness. "It didn't take very long to find the right one," she said.

Now, almost 10 years later, she is married, thinking about starting a family, and working as a professional in agriculture marketing. She and her husband, a farmer, live in an old Iowa farmhouse that they enjoy restoring.

Daiton also has learned how to live with her condition. For example, her job requires that she travel approximately 8 to 10 weeks a year all over the country. Because she knows sleepiness is an issue for her, she never drives to locations more than three hours away, always flying instead.

With medication and some helpful habits, she has her symptoms under control, and she rarely falls asleep unexpectedly. "It happens maybe once or twice a year, when I am doing something boring like data entry on my laptop," she said. "Day to day, I don't even really think about it."

For some people, sleepiness is a constant, controlling their lives and often their ability to function day to day. In this chapter we discuss two similar but different conditions that produce excessive daytime sleepiness — narcolepsy, which affects up to 50 people per 100,000 worldwide, and a less common disorder called idiopathic hypersomnia. Though they can't be cured, with treatment both conditions can be managed.

NARCOLEPSY

With narcolepsy, sleep can sweep over you without notice, even when you're doing something active. You may be talking with a friend, eating lunch or even driving your car, and you abruptly nod off, seemingly without warning. These episodes can come on so suddenly they've been given the name "sleep attacks."

Sometimes narcolepsy also causes a sudden loss of muscle tone, called cataplexy, that's commonly triggered by strong emotions, especially laughter. When cataplexy occurs, you lose the ability to control the muscles in your body for seconds or minutes, yet you remain fully conscious. Cataplexy can be localized — affecting, say, just your neck and head — or it can take hold of your entire body.

Narcolepsy is a lifelong condition. However, medicines and lifestyle changes can help you manage its symptoms. Support from others — family, friends, employers and teachers — also can help you cope with the disorder.

When boundaries become blurred
Narcolepsy is rare. The condition is thought to affect 1 in 2,000 people, but establishing how many people have it is difficult because it's often undiagnosed or mistaken for another disorder, which means a lost opportunity for treatment. It affects men and women in about equal numbers.

Narcolepsy typically appears in young people. It usually emerges during the high school years or in young adulthood. However, it can develop in children as young as 7 years old. Studies suggest that age 18 is the average age when narcolepsy symptoms appear. Occasionally people will begin seeking treatment when they're older, even in their 50s, though in some cases they've been struggling with symptoms for years.

Sleepiness and other symptoms associated with narcolepsy generally don't appear abruptly or overnight, but instead develop steadily over weeks, months or perhaps even a few years. The condition is likely to last through life, but typically it doesn't grow worse with age.

Researchers are still unraveling the causes of narcolepsy. It involves the brain's complex chemical systems that regulate wakefulness and sleepiness. With narcolepsy, neurological signaling breaks down, throwing your sleep-wake balance into chaos, fragmenting your sleep at night and extending sleepiness into your day.

When this signaling system is healthy, it helps regulate the border between dreamy rapid eye movement (REM) sleep and being awake. When the system deteriorates, the border can blur. Dreamlike hallucinations can begin to invade your daily life.

COMMON SYMPTOMS

Symptoms of narcolepsy may worsen during the first few years of the disorder, then they tend to plateau. They include excessive daytime sleepiness, sudden loss of muscle tone, changes in REM sleep, sleep paralysis and hallucinations.

This collection of symptoms can affect all parts of your day. Children and college students with the condition often find school difficult and their academic performance declines. For middle-aged and older people, functioning at work can be a challenge. Relationships can suffer, and quality of life may be affected.

Excessive daytime sleepiness
People with narcolepsy fall asleep without warning. This can happen anywhere and at any time. It can happen when you're bored or during a task. For example, you may be working or talking with friends and suddenly fall asleep. It can be especially dangerous if you fall asleep while driving.

You might fall asleep for only a few minutes or for up to a half hour. After waking, you'll often feel refreshed, but you'll get sleepy again. You also may experience a decrease in how alert and focused you feel during the day. Daytime sleepiness often is the first symptom to appear. Feeling sleepy makes it hard to focus and function.

Some people with narcolepsy continue doing a task when they fall asleep briefly. For example, you may fall asleep while writing, typing or driving. You might continue to perform that task while asleep. When you awaken, you can't remember what you did or how you got there.

Sudden loss of muscle tone
A condition in which the muscles suddenly lose their tone is called cataplexy. It can cause slurred speech or complete weakness of most

muscles that may last up to a few minutes. Not everyone with narcolepsy has this symptom.

Cataplexy is triggered by intense emotions and can't be controlled. Laughter or excitement may cause the symptoms. But sometimes fear, surprise or anger can produce loss of muscle tone, too. For example, when you laugh, your head may drop without your control. Or your knees may suddenly lose strength, causing you to fall. Some people with narcolepsy experience only one or two episodes of cataplexy a year. Others have several episodes a day.

Cataplexy can be troubling and embarrassing. One individual being treated for narcolepsy was in the middle of her wedding reception when her head flopped onto the table because a guest told a good joke. Another, a fisherman, became momentarily paralyzed and unable to move when a large fish took his bait.

Some people begin to avoid these strong, positive emotions because they don't want to be embarrassed. But that often means giving up the things that bring them the most joy.

Changes in REM sleep

With narcolepsy, REM sleep control becomes erratic. REM sleep is when most dreaming happens. Typically, people enter REM sleep 60 to 90 minutes after falling asleep. But people with narcolepsy often move more quickly to REM sleep. They tend to enter REM sleep within 15 minutes of falling asleep. REM sleep also can happen at any time of the day.

In addition, dreams that occur during REM sleep are more likely to be frightening and vivid. You may experience what are known as lucid dreams, in which you're aware that you're dreaming, and you even may be able to shape the dream narrative. Some people with narcolepsy act out their dreams.

Sleep paralysis

People with narcolepsy often experience sleep paralysis. During this state, you can't move or speak while falling asleep or upon waking. It's usually brief — lasting a few seconds or minutes. But it can be scary. You may be aware of it happening and be able to recall it afterward. Not everyone with sleep paralysis, however, has narcolepsy.

A BRIEF HISTORY OF NARCOLEPSY

In 19th-century France, a man saw a doctor because he was falling asleep repeatedly and uncontrollably, sometimes nodding off as many as 200 times a day. He couldn't stay awake for any extended period, and the man's son had to accompany him during the day to wake him up over and over again.

The doctor, whose name was Jean Baptiste Édouard Gélineau, wrote about this patient and became the first to describe this medical condition. He called it *narcolepsie*, basing the French name on the Greek words for "stupor attack."

For nearly a century the condition was poorly understood, and it was often considered a psychological illness. In the 1950s came the discovery of rapid eye movement (REM) sleep, and tests began to unveil distinct REM patterns characteristic of narcolepsy. Other tests were developed that could objectively measure sleepiness by how quickly someone dozed off for a daytime nap.

Further important work was done at Stanford University, where much of the research on the disorder has taken place. Researchers at Stanford kept and studied dogs that had narcolepsy. The dogs were discovered to have a genetic variation that caused them to have insufficient hypocretin (orexin), a brain neurotransmitter that regulates wakefulness. This discovery of a physical cause was a key breakthrough in understanding narcolepsy.

Soon it was shown that humans with narcolepsy also had low levels of this neurotransmitter or experienced abnormalities in how it functions. In the year 2000, researchers published findings that individuals with narcolepsy have 85% to 95% fewer orexin-producing nerve cells in their brains than do people who don't have narcolepsy.

Hallucinations

During sleep paralysis people sometimes see things that aren't actually there. Hallucinations also may happen in bed without sleep paralysis. These are called hypnagogic hallucinations if they happen as you fall asleep. They're called hypnopompic hallucinations if they happen upon waking. For example, you might feel as if there's a stranger in your bedroom. These hallucinations may be vivid and frightening because you may not be fully asleep when you begin dreaming.

TYPES AND CAUSES

Narcolepsy is divided into two types:
- **Type 1.** A person with type 1 narcolepsy generally experiences both excessive sleepiness and cataplexy.
- **Type 2.** An individual with type 2 narcolepsy has excessive sleepiness but not cataplexy.

Researchers aren't certain what causes narcolepsy, but they've found evidence that type 1 narcolepsy may be an autoimmune disorder in which the immune system attacks healthy cells in the body. With narcolepsy, the immune system damages brain cells that produce the hormone orexin, which helps your body stay awake.

Why the body turns on itself in this way isn't clear, but narcolepsy may involve your immune system's reaction to another infection. When narcolepsy symptoms first emerge, some people have high levels of antibodies that show a recent bacterial infection, such as from strep throat. Influenza breakouts have been shown to lead to cases of narcolepsy. Also, narcolepsy tends to emerge at the end of winter when illnesses such as flu spike. One theory is that in some people these infections trigger the immune system to attack orexin-producing cells.

Most people with type 1 narcolepsy have a variation in the genes that moderate immune reactions. This variation increases the likelihood of an immune system attack on brain cells that create orexin. Interestingly, this genetic variation is common. However, the vast majority of people who have it will never develop narcolepsy.

Researchers are still unraveling how specific genes may affect the development of narcolepsy. Generally, most people with narcolepsy don't have it in their family. However, there are some families where the condition is more common.

The loss of orexin that drives sleepiness symptoms is also thought to play a role in other symptoms, such as increasing appetite, though this isn't firmly established. People often gain weight with narcolepsy, and someone with this condition is more likely to be obese.

In type 2 narcolepsy, orexin levels remain normal, so the hormone can't be linked to its cause. For now, the cause of type 2 narcolepsy remains unknown.

DIAGNOSING NARCOLEPSY

A doctor can determine if excessive daytime sleepiness is due to narcolepsy or another sleep disorder. A diagnosis generally involves

---

SECONDARY NARCOLEPSY

Some people with a brain injury can exhibit daytime sleepiness similar to that found in narcolepsy, though there are differences between the two.

Narcolepsy associated with a brain injury is called secondary narcolepsy. It results when there's damage to the hypothalamus, a region deep inside the brain that acts as the master control of sleep. This damage may result from a tumor or disease, and it can affect the hypothalamus's ability to regulate sleep. People with secondary narcolepsy may fall asleep during the day, can sleep for long stretches or might have other neurological symptoms.

Secondary narcolepsy is usually managed by treating the underlying condition with some of the medications used to treat type 1 narcolepsy.

gathering a complete history of your symptoms, conducting a physical examination, and performing sleep studies, both at night and during the day. You also may be asked to keep a journal for 1 to 2 weeks to document your sleep and wake patterns around the clock.

A sleep study, also known as polysomnography, is one of the tests to help determine if you have narcolepsy. For this test, you must spend the night at a medical facility. The test measures your brain waves, heart rate and breathing. It also records your leg and eye movements. This data allows the medical team to track your passage through the different stages of sleep.

Individuals with narcolepsy enter REM quickly, usually within about 15 minutes of falling asleep — compared to 60 to 90 minutes for typical sleepers. A sleep study can help determine if your sleepiness is

CAN I DRIVE?

If your symptoms aren't well controlled, driving with narcolepsy can be unsafe, putting you and others at risk.

Because narcolepsy can prompt sudden sleep attacks, hallucinations or cataplexy, people with the condition have more automobile crashes and near-crashes than do people without the disorder. If you have narcolepsy, your chances of having an accident can be up to four times greater than for someone without the condition. One study found that two-thirds of people with narcolepsy had dozed off behind the wheel at some point, while nearly one-third had experienced an episode of paralysis-like cataplexy while driving.

An individual who's been diagnosed with narcolepsy is usually disqualified from holding a commercial driver's license, which is required for bus and truck drivers. However, it's possible for someone with the condition to get a license to drive a car.

When you apply for or renew a driver's license, many states will ask whether you have a medical condition that may affect

related to narcolepsy or may be caused by another condition, such as obstructive sleep apnea.

You'll also undergo a daytime exam called a multiple sleep latency test, where you're monitored while taking naps in a sleep clinic. The test measures how quickly you fall asleep and whether you enter REM sleep. People with narcolepsy fall asleep quickly during the day — often within 8 minutes — and are more likely to enter REM sleep during naps.

For a diagnosis of narcolepsy, REM sleep must come within 15 minutes during two naps in the daytime test or during one nap and nighttime sleep in the overnight sleep study.

You also may be asked questions to determine if you've experienced the near-paralysis associated with cataplexy. By one set of

your driving or cause you to lose consciousness. If the answer is yes, you may be required to get a letter from your medical provider stating that you've been evaluated and that it's safe for you to drive. In some states, such as California and Pennsylvania, medical providers are required to inform licensing officials if a person has narcolepsy.

Here are some tips to reduce the risk of an accident if you have narcolepsy and drive:
- Nap before driving.
- Don't drive for long periods.
- Keep trips short or take breaks on longer trips.
- Nap during driving breaks.
- Don't consume any alcohol before driving.
- Avoid driving after eating a meal.
- Don't drive when you might be sleepiest, such as at night.
- Don't do nighttime work that involves driving.
- Avoid emotional triggers that may bring on cataplexy.

diagnostic guidelines, this is defined as a loss of muscle tone triggered by laughter or joking, with episodes occurring at least a few times a month.

In some cases, a doctor may want to check your orexin, as levels of this wakefulness-inducing hormone are low in people with type 1 narcolepsy. However, this can't be done with a simple blood test. The test requires a spinal tap (lumbar puncture), where cerebrospinal fluid is removed with a needle that's inserted between two vertebrae in your lower back. This test is often not required to make a narcolepsy diagnosis.

Your doctor will also explore other possible causes for your excessive sleepiness. Because other sleep disorders can also produce excessive daytime sleepiness, they must be ruled out.

MANAGING NARCOLEPSY

While there's no cure for narcolepsy, the condition can be managed with medications that can help you feel more awake during the day. Lifestyle changes can help you stick to the rhythms of daily life and feel sharp and alert when you need to.

Lifestyle

Here are some simple steps that you can take to moderate the sleepiness narcolepsy brings:

- **Nap.** Schedule short naps during the times you know you will feel sleepy. This can help prevent you from falling asleep unexpectedly.
- **Maintain a healthy sleep schedule.** Go to bed and wake up close to the same time every day, and give yourself enough time in bed to get the recommended amount of sleep, which is a minimum of seven hours for most people.
- **Relax.** Make the evening a time for winding down and preparing for sleep.
- **Avoid alcohol.** Alcohol interferes with healthy sleep and should be avoided, especially in the hours before bedtime.
- **Limit caffeine.** Caffeine may help you feel awake during the day, but it can keep you from falling asleep. Avoid it in the evening.

- **Don't smoke.** Nicotine is a stimulant that interferes with sleep, and it also has many additional negative health effects. Smoking in the evening is especially harmful to sleep.
- **Exercise.** Daytime exercise can help you feel awake during the day and sleep better at night. Avoid vigorous exercise close to bedtime, as this can disturb sleep.

Medications

Medications that stimulate your nervous system can make you feel more awake during the day and help prevent you from falling asleep at unexpected times. In most cases, the last dose of a stimulant is taken at lunchtime or before 2 p.m. to prevent it from disturbing healthy nighttime sleep. Other medications can help manage the temporary paralysis of cataplexy.

It's important to tell your doctor if you're pregnant or may get pregnant. Most of the medications to treat narcolepsy can have negative effects on the baby's health or increase the risk of complications with the pregnancy.

Medications commonly prescribed for the treatment of narcolepsy include:

- **Modafinil (Provigil).** This medication helps people feel less drowsy and more alert during the day. It's sometimes referred to as a wakefulness-promoting agent because it works differently than other stimulants, such as amphetamines. This is often the first medication prescribed to treat the condition, in part because it's less addictive than other stimulants. Modafinil has been shown to reduce daytime sleepiness and improve quality of life.
- **Armodafinil (Nuvigil).** Related to modafinil, it's also considered a wakefulness-promoting agent.
- **Pitolisant (Wakix).** This drug is what's known as a histamine 3 receptor antagonist-inverse agonist. It's been shown to reduce daytime sleepiness and cataplexy. It works by increasing levels of histamine, which regulates sleep and wakefulness.
- **Sodium oxybate (Lumryz, Xyrem) and mixed-salt oxybate (Xywav).** These drugs are central nervous system depressants that can alleviate cataplexy and may improve daytime sleepiness. Because they depress the central nervous system and can slow

breathing, oxybates shouldn't be taken with alcohol, sedative hypnotics, opioids or benzodiazepines, among other medications. Oxybate medications carry a boxed warning about their potential for abuse and misuse. The medications are closely related to gamma-hydroxybutyrate (GHB), a substance that's under tight control because it's sometimes sold illegally and abused.
- **Solriamfetol (Sunosi).** It relieves excessive daytime sleepiness by increasing signaling chemicals in the brain that control wakefulness.
- **Medications containing dextroamphetamine (Dexedrine, Adderall, others) and lisdexamfetamine (Vyvanse).** These are stimulants that help many people manage excessive daytime sleepiness associated with narcolepsy.
- **Methylphenidate (Ritalin, Concerta, Quillivant XR, others).** This is an amphetamine-like stimulant that's commonly used to help people with narcolepsy stay awake and feel alert. Its effects wear off more quickly than is the case for some other stimulants.
- **Certain antidepressants.** They suppress REM sleep and can help manage cataplexy, hallucinations and sleep paralysis. However, the American Academy of Sleep Medicine found there was insufficient or inconclusive evidence to make a strong recommendation regarding their use.

IDIOPATHIC HYPERSOMNIA

Idiopathic hypersomnia is a rare condition in which people can be hit anytime by a strong need to sleep. It's not a single disease, but rather a collection of symptoms that can't be fully explained. The word *idiopathic* refers to a disease for which the cause is unknown. *Hypersomnia* refers to an inability to stay awake or alert despite adequate nighttime sleep.

Some of the symptoms of the disorder are similar to those of narcolepsy. It differs from narcolepsy, however, in that people who have it are much less likely to spontaneously fall asleep or lose muscle control due to cataplexy episodes. And while a nap may leave someone with narcolepsy feeling refreshed, at least for a short time, the same can't be said for a person with idiopathic hypersomnia. You may have difficulty waking after you've been asleep, and you may wake confused and disoriented.

Also, during sleep studies, early REM episodes aren't found with idiopathic hypersomnia — either during an overnight polysomnography or with daytime nap studies.

Treatment for the condition may include many of the same medications used to manage daytime sleepiness in narcolepsy. A stimulant medication, such as modafinil (Provigil), might be prescribed to help you stay awake during the day. Other medicines may include sodium

DO YOU NEED A 'SOCIAL PRESCRIPTION'?

Narcolepsy and idiopathic hypersomnia can be especially isolating. Symptoms such as excessive sleepiness and sleep attacks can make socializing difficult and interfere with personal and work relationships. Unfortunately, getting medical help can take a long time, and diagnosis and treatment may be delayed because of a relative shortage of sleep specialists.

However, there are ways you can begin to learn more about how to live with your sleep condition and to engage with people who are going through the same things you are. Advocacy organizations and social network groups have formed around narcolepsy and idiopathic hypersomnia, providing useful information and a sense of community. These include Wake Up Narcolepsy, Project Sleep and Narcolepsy Network. Getting involved with these groups or visiting their websites may connect you to others experiencing a similar journey, providing much-needed support.

Experts have called this a "social prescription," and emphasize that it can be an important part of living with a sleep disorder, complementing your medications, medical devices and doctor appointments. It can lead you to take an active role in managing your disorder, helping you feel better and be healthier.

oxybate (Lumryz, Xyrem), mixed-salt oxybate (Xywav), clarithromycin (Biaxin XL) and methylphenidate (Ritalin, Concerta, Quillivant XR, others).

In addition, your doctor will likely recommend healthy sleep habits such as developing a regular nighttime sleep schedule and avoiding alcohol and medications that can affect your sleep.

The same disorder?
Some sleep scientists propose that idiopathic hypersomnia and type 2 narcolepsy may represent different manifestations of the same underlying disorder, rather than two distinct conditions.

This perspective is grounded in the observation that both disorders share several key clinical features, such as excessive daytime sleepiness not relieved by adequate sleep, difficulty waking up and the absence of cataplexy. Furthermore, the fact that there's not a marked decrease in the hormone orexin brings idiopathic hypersomnia closer to that of type 2 narcolepsy. Both conditions also lack specific autoimmune markers.

Given these similarities, along with the challenges in differentiating the two conditions, sleep scientists are debating if the two conditions should be merged into one. Among other implications, such a merger could pose challenges for individuals dependent on a type 2 narcolepsy diagnosis for insurance coverage of their medications. This is because idiopathic hypersomnia frequently lacks insurance support.

The debate underscores the complexity of sleep disorders and highlights the evolving nature of sleep science as researchers strive to better characterize these conditions for improved diagnosis and treatment.

11

Restless legs syndrome

Becky had always been a good sleeper, but over the course of a year all of that changed. Some nights she doesn't sleep at all because of intense, overwhelming sensations in her legs that keep her awake.

Becky, a 76-year-old former nurse, has restless legs syndrome. Even with her medical training, she didn't appreciate how powerful the sensations could be until she felt them herself.

"Sometimes I describe it as somebody squeezing my legs," she said. "I have to move. I just have to move. There is no other way to describe it. It's awful."

Becky's story illustrates how restless legs syndrome can take a toll on your sleep and daily life, and it also exemplifies the challenges of trying to manage it.

Her symptoms began subtly. At first it was just a strange feeling at bedtime that compelled her to hang one leg over the side of the bed. Over time the feelings grew more intense and began to keep her awake for hours. Eventually the sensations grew so powerful that she was getting no sleep at all on many nights, sometimes going sleepless two nights in a row.

"I just hated the thought of bedtime because I knew I wouldn't be sleeping," she said.

To relieve the feelings, she would get out of bed and roam the house. She often ended up in the kitchen, finding she had a strong desire to eat. "I have gained about 20 pounds since this all started," she said.

Her husband of more than 50 years began sleeping in another room because of the constant disruption.

Becky finally saw her doctor. When she described the symptoms to her primary care physician, he told her that she may have restless legs syndrome. "I said, 'I don't have restless legs,'" she said. "I had always heard that restless legs was this creepy-crawly feeling, and I didn't have that. It didn't dawn on me that it was my legs."

She also admits that she held a common misperception about the condition that prevents many people from seeing their doctor. "I never thought of restless legs as anything real," she said. "I thought it was in your mind."

Like many people, Becky is finding treatment to be a constant process of trial and error, and restless legs can be particularly complicated to treat. The body can develop a tolerance to some of the medications typically used to treat the condition, and symptoms can return and even be more severe. But she's also found that by sticking with the treatment, she can improve her symptoms.

Becky was prescribed medication to treat her condition. The first medication she took worked well for a while, giving her the best night's sleep she'd had in some time. "It was wonderful," she said.

Unfortunately, after a few months, the medication was no longer effective, and the sleepless nights returned. She then tried three different medications, but they didn't deliver the results she hoped for. In the meantime, her symptoms became more intrusive, and she was now experiencing the sensations around the clock, not just at night.

Becky returned to the medication she first started taking and is seeing some improvement. She knows, though, that it may lose its effectiveness for her again.

Becky has developed other strategies to help manage her symptoms. She stands when watching TV and reading books. She often rests *the books on the kitchen counter. Long car rides remain difficult, and the last time she flew she had to stand for nearly the entire three-hour flight. At a recent conference she attended, she stood in the back so she could keep her legs moving. "It's like a little cha-cha step," she said with a laugh.*

She knows that she'll be managing this condition for the rest of her life. "I will just keep trying different stuff and see if it works."

People with restless legs syndrome often find it difficult to explain to others what they're experiencing. Words often used to describe the leg sensations include *creeping, crawling, tingling* and *antsy*, but these don't fit every case. While the condition may sound mild or insignificant, it can be terribly debilitating for those who have it.

Restless legs syndrome is considered a sleep disorder because it generally is worst at night, interfering with sleep. It's not uncommon for people who have the disorder to see a doctor because they're drained and fatigued from not being able to get a good night's rest. In addition to causing problems with sleep, the condition can have a profound impact on overall health and quality of life.

UNCONTROLLABLE URGES

Restless legs syndrome is sometimes called Willis-Ekbom disease, a nod to Sir Thomas Willis, a 17th-century London physician who was the first to describe it: "So great a Restlessness and Tossing of their Members ... that the diseased are no more able to sleep, than if they were in a Place of the greatest torture."

Today, the condition is generally defined as an urge to move your legs that worsens at night when sitting or lying down, and which is relieved only by moving the legs or getting up and walking.

By some estimates, up to 10% of the population have such urges, with about 3% experiencing moderate to severe symptoms. Women are more likely to have the condition than are men, and it tends to become much more common with age.

Symptoms of restless legs syndrome can vary widely in intensity and frequency. Some people experience relatively mild urges that appear sporadically, perhaps once a week, or even less often. This is known as intermittent restless legs syndrome. Others have them every night, and the symptoms can be overpowering. When symptoms are more severe and occur at least twice a week, the condition is known as chronic persistent restless legs syndrome.

With either condition, the urge to move becomes uncontrollable, and the only way to relieve the symptoms is to get up and walk. Because of this, sleep can become nearly impossible some nights. Symptoms of the condition also can take a toll on mood, the ability to concentrate, memory and productivity.

But despite the impact it can have, it's not uncommon for restless legs syndrome to be overlooked by medical professionals and to go undiagnosed.

In this chapter, we'll explain what scientists have learned about the cause of restless legs syndrome and how doctors diagnose the condition. We'll also share some practical tips that may bring positive effects right away, as well as discuss the benefits and limitations of medications used to treat the condition. Managing restless legs isn't always easy, and it's best done in close consultation with your doctor or a sleep specialist. But chances are good that, working together, you can reduce the urges causing you so much discomfort and fatigue.

POSSIBLE CAUSES

Researchers don't fully understand what causes restless legs syndrome, though they've uncovered many clues. Factors thought to be involved include genetics, iron deficiency and irregularities in the action of certain brain chemicals.

Dopamine

A leading suspect in the development of restless legs syndrome is dopamine, a brain neurotransmitter that helps regulate the signals your body sends to move your muscles. In people with the condition, this signaling system may no longer work properly, even if dopamine levels are normal.

While scientists don't fully understand how this dysfunction leads to an overwhelming urge to move your legs, there's plenty of evidence pointing to dopamine as a likely cause. For instance, dopamine levels naturally fall in the evening and at night, which is when symptoms typically arise. In addition, some medicines that do reduce the disturbing leg sensations associated with restless legs syndrome work by stimulating dopamine receptors.

Iron deficiency
Many people with restless legs syndrome have low iron levels in the part of the brain responsible for movement. However, the role of iron as a cause of restless legs syndrome might be indirect and lead back to dopamine.

Iron is essential for the brain to process dopamine and enable the neurotransmitter to function correctly. Low iron levels may be preventing dopamine from doing its job. In some cases, restoring iron levels can reduce symptoms.

Iron deficiency is extremely common during pregnancy, and, therefore, it's not unusual for restless legs syndrome to develop then. Hormonal changes also may be involved.

Genetics
Your genes may play a part in restless legs syndrome, though it's not yet fully understood exactly how. What is clear is that you're more likely to develop the condition if you have a close relative who has it. More than half of people with restless legs syndrome have a family member who has the condition. When symptoms appear early in life, there's thought to be a genetic factor involved.

In the past two decades, researchers have discovered several genes associated with restless legs syndrome. Variations in some of these genes can lead to irregular iron levels, suggesting to some researchers that this may be the link to restless legs syndrome. Other genetic variations relate to how your body metabolizes dopamine. These genetic variations may be passed down from parents to their children.

Genetic variations alone, however, may not cause restless legs syndrome. Researchers believe something else triggers the onset of symptoms. In addition to an iron deficiency, possible triggers may include kidney dysfunction and cardiovascular disease, though the connection to cardiovascular disease is less clear.

Taking antidepressant medications may potentially trigger the onset of symptoms or make them worse. One antidepressant that doesn't appear to aggravate symptoms is bupropion (Wellbutrin), which is

DOPAMINE: A SOURCE OF PLEASURE AND DISCOMFORT

Dopamine is often referred to as the pleasure hormone because it's associated with your brain's reward system, a network of structures responsible for pleasure, motivation and reinforcement. The hormone also may be involved in the development of unpleasurable sensations. Dopamine is the leading suspect behind the anguishing symptoms of restless legs syndrome.

Both a hormone and a brain chemical messenger (neurotransmitter), dopamine plays multiple roles, using different pathways to send signals that keep your body's systems running smoothly. One of those pathways involves the brain's reward center. Exercise and sex, for example, can increase dopamine levels, bringing pleasure or making you feel better. The hormone is also involved with sleep, eating, thinking, learning, smell, vision and, importantly, muscle movement.

Movement is controlled by a part of the brain called the basal ganglia, which requires certain levels of dopamine to function normally. When those levels drop too low or climb too high, movement can become uncontrolled or uncoordinated. For example, people who have Parkinson's disease can lose some control of movement because the neurons involved with dopamine signaling in this part of the brain have degenerated and lost some of their functionality.

Scientists continue to explore dopamine's involvement in restless legs syndrome, but research as to a specific cause remains inconclusive.

sometimes recommended for people with restless legs syndrome who take an antidepressant. The relationship between restless legs syndrome and antidepressants is being challenged, however, and it remains unclear to what extent these medications may exacerbate the condition. Other medications that may aggravate symptoms include some antipsychotic drugs, some anti-nausea medications and some cold and allergy medicines.

Studies also suggest that caffeine, nicotine, alcohol, stress or too little exercise may worsen symptoms.

DIAGNOSING RESTLESS LEGS SYNDROME

There's no definitive test or imaging technology that can detect restless legs syndrome. Instead, your doctor or a sleep specialist will likely ask you questions to help determine if you experience the telltale symptoms of the condition.

Sometimes blood tests may be conducted to reveal potential conditions that may be contributing to the problem. If your iron levels are low, for example, your symptoms may improve with medications to boost iron.

Guidelines commonly used to diagnose restless legs syndrome include five criteria. You must have all five before you can be diagnosed with the condition. These are:
1. You feel an urge to move your legs, which may or may not be accompanied by other uncomfortable sensations in your legs.
2. The urge begins or worsens when you're resting or inactive, such as when sitting or lying down.
3. Symptoms are relieved when you move your legs.
4. Symptoms worsen at night.
5. No other medical condition or behavior is causing the symptoms.

There's a handy mnemonic device for remembering key symptoms of the disorder — just spell URGE. The U stands for an uncontrollable urge to move; R is for rest, because the urge appears when you rest; G indicates that the symptoms get better with movement; and E means symptoms appear or get worse in the evening.

Common tests

As part of the diagnostic process, you might be asked to complete a questionnaire to help identify the severity and frequency of your symptoms. This questionnaire typically asks you to rate your level of discomfort, the strength of your urges to move and the amount of relief you get from moving. You also may be asked how often you get symptoms and how much they affect your sleep and feelings of being rested during the day, as well as their impact on your mood and daily life.

Be prepared to answer these questions:
- How often do you have these urges to move? How long do they last? How intense are they?
- Does moving relieve these feelings?
- Are the urges painful?
- How long does it take you to fall asleep?
- Are you sleepy during the day?

Among other things, the questionnaire can help determine if you have the intermittent form of the disorder or the chronic form. This information can be important in determining how to treat your condition.

Sometimes a doctor will request a sleep study (see page 196). The test can't diagnose restless legs syndrome, but it can provide additional information about your overall sleep health and whether you have something called periodic limb movement disorder, which is often associated with restless legs syndrome. Periodic limb movement is a sleep disorder characterized by repetitive movements of the legs and feet during sleep. Most, but not all, people who have restless legs syndrome also experience periodic limb movements during sleep.

Once a diagnosis has been made, work can begin on a plan to treat the condition. A bit of patience will serve you well because treatment can take time to show results.

TREATMENT

The goal of treatment is to reduce your symptoms and improve your quality of life. Some treatments for restless legs syndrome can take time to work, but there are several things that you can do on your own that may help right away.

As you and your doctor consider treatment options, it's important to evaluate how much of an impact the condition is having on your life. You might think of this as an assessment of your "misery factor," and the higher your misery factor is, the more aggressive you may want to be with treatment. If you're bothered just a couple of times a month and moving around for a few minutes brings your symptoms under control, home remedies may be sufficient. But if you find yourself up and pacing nearly every night, unable to sleep, you may want to try medication to see if it can help.

Lifestyle changes
Lifestyle changes and self-care strategies are often a good first step. Many people find they can lessen the symptoms of restless legs syndrome with some simple steps they take at home. For mild symptoms that appear occasionally, this may be all the treatment needed. With moderate or severe symptoms, these steps can boost the effectiveness of other treatments, such as medications.

Massage
Gentle leg massage not only is relaxing but also provides something called counterstimulation. To understand how this works, let's think of another common example of counterstimulation: If you hit your thumb with a hammer, you may stick your thumb in your mouth to make it feel better. There's no medicine in your mouth, of course, but sucking your thumb stimulates the nerves around the site of the injury and creates a sort of sensory overload that helps obscure the pain.

In the same way, stimulating nerves in your legs with massage, pressure or vibration gives some people relief by making their urge sensations less noticeable.

Limit or avoid caffeine, alcohol and tobacco
Reducing or eliminating these substances may relieve symptoms. Keep in mind that the closer to bedtime you consume them, the more likely it is that they may contribute to your symptoms.

Stretching and exercise before bed
Ten minutes of stretching before bed can be a big help for some. Exercise helps reduce symptoms, and it increases dopamine levels. Any heart-pumping cardio workouts should be done earlier in the day, but a stroll in the evening may help minimize symptoms at bedtime.

Pedaling
Some people with restless legs find that they can more easily sit in one place if they pedal while they sit. To do this, you can use a relatively simple device that's placed in front of a chair. The device consists of two pedals within a small rack. Some people pedal on a stationary bike with the resistance set on low.

Warm bath, massage and socks
Soaking in a warm bath and massaging your legs may relieve symptoms by relaxing your muscles. Some people also find that putting on warm socks or compression stockings and wearing them to bed helps.

Heating pads or ice packs
Applying either heat or cold to your legs may reduce symptoms. Some people find greater relief with heating pads, while others prefer ice packs. You might even try alternating between warm and cold.

Stress
Do what you can to manage stress. Data suggests that stress can increase restless legs symptoms, and relieving stress may reduce them.

Sleep habits
You might begin by keeping to a regular sleep schedule — going to bed and getting up at nearly the same time each day. Also, try to get 7 to 8 hours of sleep each night. Good sleep habits form a strong foundation for your other treatments to work better.

Medications
Depending on the results of your diagnostic tests and how well home remedies work for you, your doctor might recommend iron supplements or prescription medications as part of your treatment.

The Food and Drug Administration (FDA) has approved only a few medications specifically for treatment of restless legs syndrome. However, other medications, including some that were developed to treat conditions such as Parkinson's disease, also have been found to be effective for restless legs syndrome. These medications are prescribed off-label, a common practice.

But don't expect all your symptoms to disappear. Medications generally don't cure restless legs syndrome, but they may provide noticeable relief. As you set your expectations for treatment, consider a goal of reducing your symptoms by about 75% — in some cases the results may be better and in others not as good.

It may take several trials to find the right medication or combination of medications that works best for you. Also, most medications used to treat restless legs syndrome aren't recommended if you're pregnant.

Iron therapy

Symptoms of restless legs syndrome may be associated with low iron stores in a part of the brain involved with movement. Blood tests allow your doctor to look for evidence of low iron stores. These tests commonly include one for iron in your blood and another for ferritin, a protein that stores iron in tissues in the body.

If the tests suggest your iron stores may be low, your doctor might recommend iron replacement therapy on a trial basis for at least three months to see if your symptoms improve. Even when iron supplements prove effective, they can take some time to work, and it may be weeks or months before you begin to notice results.

In some cases, oral iron supplements can bring marked improvement to restless legs syndrome and no other medications are needed. Generally, though, improvement is more modest.

While iron supplements are available for sale over the counter at your pharmacy or grocery store, don't take them unless your doctor recommends it. It's possible to get too much iron through supplements. Eating iron-rich foods, such as green leafy vegetables, however, is always a good idea.

Iron supplements are often taken with vitamin C, which helps your body absorb the iron. A typical dose is 325 milligrams (mg) of the supplement ferrous sulfate and 100 to 200 mg of vitamin C, taken on an empty stomach. Your doctor might recommend that you take the supplements at night because some studies have shown iron is absorbed by the brain most effectively then.

Some individuals find that iron supplements can cause considerable stomach upset or that they don't absorb the iron through the gut. In these cases, the medications may be given intravenously. This can also speed up the time it takes for the treatment to show results, leading to improvement in symptoms in 2 to 4 weeks.

Gabapentin, pregabalin and gabapentin enacarbil

The drug gabapentin (Neurontin, Gralise) is often one of the first to be prescribed for restless legs syndrome. This medication and ones similar to it were developed to treat seizures. The medications bind with a specific protein in cells, altering the way brain neurotransmitters are released.

Gabapentin was approved to treat epilepsy in the 1990s. Since then, it and similar medications have become widely prescribed for several other conditions, including restless legs syndrome. Although few large studies have been conducted, decades of experience show that the medication improves symptoms of restless legs syndrome in many people.

Gabapentin is commonly taken 1 to 2 hours before symptoms typically begin. You'll likely start with a very low dose and increase the dosage gradually until it becomes effective. When high doses are required to relieve symptoms, the medication is sometimes taken in small amounts throughout the day for better absorption. It's important that you take the medication as your doctor recommends or it may produce adverse effects or not work as intended.

A related medication, called gabapentin enacarbil (Horizant), received FDA approval for treating restless legs syndrome after studies found it to be effective for reducing symptoms. It's more easily absorbed than gabapentin and is converted into gabapentin within the body.

Another similar medication, pregabalin (Lyrica), may also be effective in relieving symptoms of restless legs syndrome, but with potentially fewer side effects.

Side effects of these drugs may include drowsiness and dizziness, which can impair driving and increase the risk of falls. However, when the dose is initially low and built up gradually, most people tolerate the medications very well.

Dopamine medications
These drugs relieve symptoms of restless legs syndrome by increasing levels of the chemical messenger dopamine, or they mimic the way it works in the brain to control movement. Because of potentially serious adverse effects, dopamine medications are typically recommended only after gabapentin or related drugs have failed to reduce symptoms.

Use of dopamine medications for restless legs syndrome goes back decades. A combination of two drugs, carbidopa and levodopa, was approved to treat Parkinson's disease in the mid-1970s, and people soon found it also brought relief for restless legs syndrome. Because the medication increases levels of dopamine, its effectiveness in reducing restless legs symptoms fueled the theory that the condition results from a disruption in how dopamine is processed in the brain.

By the 1990s, carbidopa-levodopa became a preferred treatment for restless legs syndrome, but a significant side effect began to emerge. Approximately 80% of people who took the medication regularly found that their symptoms improved for a time but then returned. And when the symptoms came back, they were often more severe and frequent than they had been originally, a phenomenon called augmentation. Symptoms that had previously appeared only at night began to show up earlier in the evening, and people who had symptoms in the evening began to have them in the afternoon. In some cases, people began having symptoms around the clock.

Because of the risk of augmentation, carbidopa-levodopa (Duopa, Sinemet, others) is now typically prescribed only if you have restless legs symptoms infrequently and don't need to take the medication every day. It can also benefit people who have restless legs only in specific, limited situations, such as long car rides or airplane flights.

The FDA has approved several medications that treat restless legs syndrome by mimicking dopamine. They include rotigotine (Neupro), delivered through an extended-release skin patch you apply each day, and pramipexole (Mirapex ER) and ropinirole, each of which comes in a pill to be taken in the hours before bedtime. These medications also may lead to symptoms returning and worsening, though this may be less frequent than with some other drugs. The extent to which this happens with the rotigotine patch may be less frequent.

> **DOPAMINE MEDICATIONS AND RISKY BEHAVIORS**
>
> Medications that affect dopamine levels can make people more likely to act in a risky manner, sometimes with severe consequences. When the behavior becomes frequent, it may be diagnosed as an impulse control disorder.
>
> In one well-known study, individuals with restless legs syndrome who took a dopamine medication for several months had an increased likelihood of developing problems related to compulsive gambling and compulsive shopping, along with other destructive behaviors. The study concluded that nearly 1 in 6 people treated with dopamine medications will develop impulse control disorders.
>
> For some individuals, loss of impulse control can lead to devastating outcomes. The study included real stories of people who began doing unusual things while taking the medications, including a woman who had never gambled before but began losing $6,000 per month on slot machines; an elderly man who bought cars and a penthouse for girlfriends; a woman who spent $5,000 on a television shopping channel; and a man who began binge eating and spending hours watching pornography on the internet.
>
> Medications that boost dopamine levels in the part of the brain involved with movement also can affect the brain's reward system and the ability to control impulses. If you or a family member or friend are taking a medication that alters dopamine levels and you notice signs of increased risky behavior, contact a doctor right away.

Opioids

Medications to treat restless legs syndrome don't bring relief for everyone. When medication and lifestyle changes fail to relieve severe, debilitating symptoms, a doctor may prescribe opioids. These medications are generally taken under the close supervision of a sleep specialist.

Opioids need to be used with great care because of side effects such as constipation or nausea, as well as risk of dependence. Tramadol (ConZip), a lower-potency opioid, is sometimes prescribed for restless legs syndrome at the smallest possible dose needed to produce results. In some very severe cases, such as those where symptoms last all day, more potent forms of the medication are sometimes prescribed.

Sleeping pills

Because sleep can be so difficult to get when your legs are restless, you might wonder if sleep aids can help. Generally, sleeping pills aren't effective at improving symptoms of restless legs syndrome, though in some cases they might play a role in treatment.

When restless legs syndrome also causes insomnia, some people find sleep medications can help them sleep. However, for many others, sleep aids can make things worse. It's as if the urges from restless legs are stronger than the sleeping pills, leaving people feeling both sleepy and wide awake at the same time, as well as overwhelmed by the sensations in their limbs.

If you have trouble sleeping because of restless legs syndrome, it's usually best to concentrate on treating the symptoms, and sleep improvements will usually follow.

A class of drugs known as benzodiazepines, which include the medications clonazepam and lorazepam, may be prescribed for a short period to help people with restless legs sleep. However, these drugs have several adverse side effects, including risk of dependence.

Devices

The FDA has approved some medical devices for treating restless legs syndrome that are available by prescription.

One is a simple cloth and foam device with pressure pads that uses a Velcro wrap to hold the pads in place. When worn in the evening, it applies pressure to your foot, which is intended to relieve symptoms of restless legs. A small six-week study done by the manufacturer found that 27 of the 30 people who used the wrap experienced an improvement in symptoms.

Another device uses mechanical vibration, with the goal of improving sleep through counterstimulation. The idea is that your nerves become busy responding to the vibrations and can't produce restless sensations. The device, which is placed under your legs, consists of a foam pad with six small motors that vibrate. You use it while you're trying to fall asleep, and it turns itself off after 35 minutes. Two small studies indicated a modest improvement in symptoms.

PREGNANCY AND RESTLESS LEGS

Restless legs syndrome during pregnancy is common. About 1 in 4 pregnant women experience the condition, which often emerges in the final trimester. In severe cases, it can contribute to complications in the pregnancy.

Researchers don't fully understand why pregnancy leads to restless legs symptoms. One theory is that symptoms are driven by the change in hormones, including estrogen, progesterone and prolactin. However, this theory isn't fully supported by research.

Another theory suggests that a decrease in levels of iron and other nutrients contributes to symptoms. Blood volume increases during pregnancy, diluting levels of iron, which is needed for dopamine to properly regulate physical movement. Similarly, pregnancy can also bring a decrease in folic acid, another important nutrient involved with dopamine. Some researchers believe that dopamine becomes disrupted because of the reduction of these nutrients. One shortcoming of this theory is that once the child is born, symptoms of restless legs often disappear before iron and folic acid levels return to normal.

The latest device to receive FDA approval is a cuff worn just beneath the knee. It supplies subtle electrical impulses to stimulate nerves in the legs. According to the manufacturer, the impulses activate muscles in the lower legs to "mimic the sensation of movement." One study found that the device did reduce symptoms for most people.

COPING AND SUPPORT

Restless legs syndrome is generally a lifelong condition. Developing coping strategies is important. They can help you to manage the

---

Likewise, pregnancy can lead to a decrease in vitamin D, which is also necessary for dopamine to be effective.

Many of the medications used to treat restless legs syndrome shouldn't be used during pregnancy. In cases when symptoms are especially severe, a medication may sometimes be prescribed in the last trimester of pregnancy. Boosting iron levels is often part of treatment for the condition.

Lifestyle measures such as massage, yoga and moderate exercise are often recommended to help reduce symptoms. Warm baths, however, should be kept short because high temperatures can cause complications in the pregnancy.

In most cases the symptoms will go away after childbirth. However, it's possible the symptoms will eventually return. Women who experience symptoms of restless legs during pregnancy are four times more likely to develop the condition later in life.

CHILDREN WITH RESTLESS LEGS

About 2% to 4% of children develop restless legs syndrome. The percentage is believed to be significantly higher in families where a parent has the condition.

As in adults, the disorder is characterized by an irresistible urge to move the legs, usually accompanied by uncomfortable sensations. These sensations typically occur in the evening or nighttime hours when the child is resting or lying down and can significantly impair the child's ability to fall asleep or stay asleep.

Diagnosing restless legs syndrome in children can be difficult because often they aren't able to communicate their symptoms clearly. In addition, the condition is often misdiagnosed, with symptoms frequently attributed to attention-deficit/hyperactivity disorder (ADHD). Complicating the matter, many children with ADHD also have restless legs symptoms. The two conditions, however, are distinct. In some cases, restless legs in children is mistakenly attributed to growing pains. However, growing pains don't cause a constant urge to move, a characteristic of restless legs syndrome.

Among children, restless legs syndrome is usually managed by improving sleep routines, limiting caffeine and increasing exercise, among other lifestyle changes.

If your child is having difficulty sleeping, it's important to see a medical professional for further evaluation and to determine the exact cause of their symptoms.

Another condition that can affect children is a newly identified sleep disorder called restless sleep disorder. It's characterized by significant restlessness during sleep, which leads to impaired daytime functioning. Children with restless sleep disorder often frequently toss and turn during the night, have difficulty maintaining a peaceful state of sleep and exhibit large body movements. During the day, symptoms often include fatigue, mood disturbances or problems with attention and behavior.

disorder and live better with its symptoms. Here are some strategies to consider:

- **Tell others about your condition.** Sharing information about restless legs syndrome will help your family members, friends and co-workers better understand when they see you pacing the halls, standing at the back of the theater or walking to the watercooler many times throughout the day.
- **Don't resist your need for movement.** If you attempt to suppress the urge to move, you may find that your symptoms only worsen. Gentle stretching or taking a walk can both reduce symptoms in the moment and keep them at bay.
- **Keep a sleep diary.** Keep track of treatment strategies that help and those that don't. Share this information with your doctor.
- **Stretch and massage.** Begin and end your day with stretching exercises or a gentle massage.
- **Seek help.** Support groups bring together individuals with restless legs as well as family members. By participating in a support group, your insights not only can help you but also may help someone else. Plus, it can be comforting to talk to others who share your experiences.

12

Unusual behaviors during sleep

Steve's nights were anything but typical. Caught in a state of limbo between sleep and wakefulness, he would get out of bed, head toward the kitchen and begin searching through the cupboards and refrigerator. His middle-of-the-night treks were spurred not so much by hunger as by what he calls "this crazy drive to get up and eat."

Steve was especially drawn to sugary foods, though he didn't usually crave these during the day. In the middle of the night, he would eat bowls of cereal, dishes of ice cream, and leftover cake or other sweets. His wife grew concerned.

Steve, a retired Lutheran minister, says that during his kitchen raids he felt as if he was both asleep and awake at the same time. The next day he usually was able to remember what happened the night before. But he felt like he couldn't control what he was doing, and it left him embarrassed and ashamed.

Desperate to halt the nighttime food binges, Steve went so far as to install padlocks on the refrigerators and the kitchen cupboards in the couple's home and their lake house. And he gave his wife the keys.

Steve has what's called a sleep-related eating disorder, an unusual behavior that occurs when a person is in a state of both wakefulness and sleep. Like many people with this type of disorder, Steve also has restless legs syndrome. Together, the conditions have taken a toll on the quality of his sleep, and he finds himself feeling tired during the day. "I feel like a dud," he said.

After finally seeing a sleep specialist, Steve learned that his sleep disorder can be managed, and his symptoms have improved. Under the care of a sleep physician, Steve is taking medications to treat both his eating disorder and his restless legs. Steve says the results have been good.

He's also made lifestyle adjustments. While sweets are locked in a cupboard at night, he can get bananas in the kitchen anytime he wants. On those nights he finds himself in the kitchen half asleep at 2 a.m. with a drive to eat, a healthy banana will usually satisfy him, and he heads back to bed.

Steve also goes for long walks in the Arizona desert, covering many miles a day. He says the movement soothes him and relieves some of his symptoms. As something of a joke, he's given himself the nickname "Fireball" to counter the fatigue he often experiences.

For many people with behaviors like Steve's, finding the right treatment often requires patience to determine the approach that's most helpful. And while treatment can reduce the disorder's negative impact, the condition can't be cured.

Steve knows he'll have to continue managing his sleep conditions for the rest of his life, but his daily hikes help him remain upbeat about the future. "I am captivated by the imagery of the cactus that is starting to blossom, and that gives me peace and hope," he said.

In the deepest parts of their sleep, some people get out of bed and do unusual things. Their eyes are wide open, though they may appear glassy-eyed or confused. If you say something to them, they likely won't respond. If they seem to be both asleep and awake, they indeed are.

Sleepwalking is one of the most common types of parasomnias, a group of conditions that includes a wide range of unwanted, sometimes bizarre behaviors that occur when you're sleeping, falling asleep or waking up. Parasomnias may be triggered by a disturbance in sleep or occur during periods of transition, such as when entering or coming out of a deep sleep.

Parasomnias range from the relatively benign tendency to mumble or moan in the night to extremely dangerous activities, such as driving while partly asleep or striking a bed partner while acting out a nightmare. With one type of parasomnia, people go to the kitchen and binge eat, usually fatty, sugary foods but sometimes inedible or toxic substances that can be harmful. Other parasomnias can prompt a person to sit bolt upright in bed, confused and disoriented, or, with yet another condition, to be inconsolably terrified, their face locked in an expression of horror.

The list of things people do while partly asleep is as strange as it is long. One study of parasomnias cataloged activities that were not much different from what a person would do while awake, such as looking at a mobile phone or turning on the light. Other behaviors were more elaborate, including making a meal, packing a suitcase or doing laundry.

In some cases the actions were inexplicable and irrational, such as taking a door off its hinges or cutting an electric cord with scissors. Some people injured themselves, breaking bones, dislocating joints or cutting themselves so severely that they needed stitches. At times people described their actions as violent, posing a risk not just to themselves but to others.

From the outside, parasomnias can be a confusing jumble of unusual behaviors. Experts have differentiated these by their causes and symptoms and sorted them into several categories. Some occur after something disturbs your sleep, but you don't complete the transition from being asleep to being awake. Some occur only during rapid eye movement (REM) sleep, while others take place only during non-REM sleep. Adding one more complication, a person can behave abnormally in both REM and non-REM sleep, where parasomnias overlap.

Understanding the different types of parasomnias can be the first step toward determining what is happening and what treatment may be most appropriate.

DISORDERS OF AROUSAL

We tend to think of being asleep and being awake as clearly defined, mutually exclusive states — you're in either one or the other. However, sometimes the boundaries blur, and you can be in varying levels of sleep and wakefulness at the same time.

Some parasomnias take place when something disturbs you during deep sleep and arouses you. As you come out of deep sleep, your brain fails to go through every process needed to wake you, and you end up in competing states of consciousness, part awake and part asleep. The parts of your brain that allow you to walk and do basic activities are awake, but the parts that help you think clearly, exercise judgment and remember events remain in a state of sleep.

When sleep disruptions frequently push you into this dual state of sleep and wakefulness, it's called a disorder of arousal. Because these disorders usually are related to a transition from the non-REM stages of sleep, particularly deep sleep, they're sometimes called non-REM sleep disorders. This differentiates them from disorders related to REM sleep, which often include dreaming.

Among individuals with a tendency to experience parasomnias, anything that increases deep sleep can raise the chances of having an episode. This can include sleep deprivation, certain medications, emotional stress or a fever or other illness. This also helps explain why parasomnia episodes are most likely in the first half of the night, because that's when most deep sleep occurs. It may not take much of a disturbance to trigger an episode. It can be a noise or another sleep condition, such as obstructive sleep apnea.

There are several disorders of arousal, with sleepwalking being the best known. All have a genetic component and can be triggered by a lack of sleep and other types of physical and mental stress.

SLEEPWALKING

Sleepwalking (somnambulism) can be dangerous or destructive. Someone who sleepwalks may leave the bedroom or even the house. They may do inexplicable and possibly harmful things, such as urinating in a closet, stepping off a balcony, falling down the stairs, injuring themselves with a knife in the kitchen, shooting a gun or driving a car. In rare cases, a sleepwalker can be physically aggressive and injure a bed partner or family member. It's important to seek prompt medical attention for violent behaviors.

Sleepwalking is most common among the very young, affecting more than 1 in 6 children. It can be considered a normal part of a child's development, peaking between the ages of 8 and 12 years. Most children will grow out of the disorder. Children who sleepwalk are also likely to talk in their sleep and experience sleep terrors.

Sleepwalking is less common after adolescence; it's estimated to affect 4% of adults. Genetics are thought to play a role in sleepwalking, and you're more likely to display this behavior if one or both of your parents were sleepwalkers.

You may be unable to wake someone who's sleepwalking, but if you do, that person is likely to be very confused. An awakened sleep-

---

SLEEPING PILLS AND UNUSUAL BEHAVIORS

Some sleep medications have been closely associated with an increase in sleepwalking and other unusual behaviors, sometimes with tragic results.

In 2019, the Food and Drug Administration (FDA) required pharmaceutical companies to add a warning to certain sleeping pills about an increased risk of unusual and possibly dangerous activities, known as complex sleep behaviors.

This "boxed warning," the most severe the agency can require, is mandatory on packaging for zolpidem (Ambien, Edluar, Zolpimist, others), eszopiclone (Lunesta) and zaleplon (Sonata). Together, these medications are sometimes referred to as the Z-drugs. Zolpidem in particular is often linked to these unusual behaviors, in part because it's so widely used, taken by more than 2.4 million people in the United States.

walker typically will be deeply disoriented and have no memory of the episode. In some cases, the confusion can cause the person to become violent.

What's happening?
Sleepwalking occurs when something disturbs you during deep sleep but fails to awaken you completely. Anything that increases either deep sleep or disturbances to sleep can trigger an episode among individuals who are prone to sleepwalk.

In adults, sleepwalking may be prompted by sleep deprivation, stress or fever. Or it may be related to another sleep disorder that disrupts sleep, such as obstructive sleep apnea. It's often associated with restless legs syndrome.

Sleepwalking episodes may be brought on by medications used to treat sleep or psychiatric disorders. Zolpidem (Ambien) is a widely used sleep aid that has frequently been associated with an increase in

---

The FDA mandated the label warning after learning that over 26 years, certain sleep medications led to 66 cases of complex sleep behaviors resulting in injury or death.

The medications are sedatives that suppress your ability to wake up. Because many unusual behaviors occur when you don't fully awaken after being disturbed, sleep medications increase the odds that you may slip into a state of being half asleep and half awake.

Contact your doctor immediately if you take one of these sleep medications and have experienced any indications of unusual behavior during sleep, such as sleepwalking or doing things you don't remember.

sleepwalking and other unusual behaviors during sleep. Some antidepressants, mood stabilizers, anti-seizure medications and antipsychotics also have been associated with sleepwalking. Because it fragments sleep, alcohol may be a trigger as well.

Frequent sleepwalking can often have serious consequences for the sleepwalker and for those around them, and it requires medical attention. If you believe you or a loved one is at risk because of sleepwalking, discuss it with your doctor. An occasional episode of mild sleepwalking, however, may not warrant seeing a doctor, though you should mention it at your next appointment.

Under any circumstances, take precautions to reduce the risk of injury from potential dangers, including falling down the stairs, tripping on toys or furniture, or tumbling out an open window. Alarms are available that will sound if you get out of bed or pass through a door.

If you see a doctor, you may be asked to complete a sleep diary for a week or two, as well as provide a detailed medical history, including medications and drug use. You may be asked to undergo an overnight sleep study in a sleep clinic to reveal more about your sleep patterns.

In some cases, a doctor may find another condition, such as obstructive sleep apnea, that's fragmenting your sleep, leading to sleepwalking. Managing that condition may end the sleepwalking. Treatment might also involve changing a medication that may be contributing to the problem.

Because sleep deprivation can lead to sleepwalking, getting a good night's sleep may reduce the frequency of episodes. Establish a sleep routine with a set schedule that allows you to get a full night's sleep.

SLEEP-RELATED EATING DISORDER

Eating while not fully awake is known as sleep-related eating disorder. The condition is frequently related to sleepwalking, but a person with this disorder has a driving desire to eat during sleep. Often there's a craving for unhealthy, high-calorie foods. During an episode, you may be attracted to syrup, peanut butter or other sugary or fatty foods, even if you don't typically like them. Weight gain is inevitable.

People who eat while asleep may prepare food quickly, using knives and the stove recklessly, and fire is a real danger. Or they may not prepare the food at all and instead eat something such as raw bacon or raw ground beef. People have even been known to eat coffee grounds, buttered cigarette butts and, even more perilously, toxic cleaning solutions.

Some people with a sleep-related eating disorder say the drive to eat can't be compared to simply being hungry and that it's best described as an overwhelming compulsion.

In the morning, the individual often won't remember the episode. In some instances, though, they may wake while bingeing, finish what they're eating and then head back to bed. People who do recall an episode often describe it as being "half awake" or "half asleep." As with sleepwalking, the eating episodes usually occur in the first few hours of sleep and after you've been aroused during non-REM sleep.

Though rare, the condition is more common among people who also have an eating disorder. Women are more likely than men to have the condition, which often appears when they are in their 20s.

What's happening?

Sleep-related eating disorders are sometimes associated with other sleep disorders, most notably restless legs syndrome. Small studies have found that more than one-third of people being treated for restless legs syndrome also had sleep-related eating disorder. Treating restless legs symptoms may reduce or eliminate the sleep-related eating disorder. In some cases, though, restless legs syndrome is misdiagnosed as insomnia, and a prescription is given for sleep medication that may inadvertently bring on symptoms of sleep-related eating disorder.

Several other sleep disorders are also associated with sleep-related eating disorder, including obstructive sleep apnea, periodic limb movement disorder, narcolepsy and some circadian rhythm disorders. In addition, the condition may have a genetic component. In one well-documented case, a man had the condition, as did his fraternal twin daughters.

Certain medications are frequently associated with sleep-related eating disorder, including hypnotic sleep aids such as zolpidem

(Ambien) and medications used to treat mental health disorders, including serotonin-norepinephrine reuptake inhibitors and psychostimulants.

If you binge eat during sleep, seek medical care. Your doctor will likely gather a detailed medical history, including a list of medications you take and any other substances you use. You may be asked to complete a sleep diary cataloging your sleep patterns. You also may be asked to undergo an overnight sleep study to determine if other sleep disorders are contributing to your symptoms. Your doctor may request that you bring along some of the foods you typically binge on at night so that you can eat them during the night in the clinic.

If your doctor finds that another sleep disorder is contributing to your symptoms, treatment may be directed at that problem first. Your doctor might also change your medications if they may be leading to the nightly binges.

Safety is a paramount concern. It's important to keep a clear path from the bedroom to the kitchen. You may also want to make items such as knives inaccessible.

Sleep-related eating disorder shouldn't be confused with a different condition that also involves nighttime eating, called nocturnal eating syndrome. With nocturnal eating syndrome, a person is awake and usually can't sleep because of hunger. They may go to the kitchen and binge eat, consuming high-calorie foods. Some consume more than one-third of their daily total calorie intake at night, often resulting in weight gain. This condition, too, requires medical care.

CONFUSIONAL AROUSALS AND SLEEP TERRORS

Some people, especially children, can become outwardly confused and disoriented during sleep. They may sit up in bed, anxious and unsettled, and in some ways appear to be awake, though they may not respond if you speak to them. This is called confusional arousal, and, like sleepwalking, it occurs when a disturbance fails to wake a person completely from deep sleep.

A similar though more dramatic condition is known as sleep terrors. During a sleep terror, your child might sit up in bed suddenly with a scream or yell. They may look wide-eyed and scared and may be breathing hard. You may not be able to wake your child, and if you do, they may be confused and inconsolable. These episodes will usually pass after 15 minutes or less but sometimes can go on for an hour.

What's happening?
A sleep terror isn't the same as a nightmare. With a nightmare, you're asleep during the frightening dream and then wake up, the fear and

---

HOW TO HANDLE CHILDHOOD SLEEP TERRORS OR SLEEPWALKING

Sleep terrors and sleepwalking aren't uncommon in children. However, seeing a child sitting up in bed in the grip of fear can be almost as terrifying for the parent, and it can be difficult to know what to do.

Here are some tips on how to respond to your child's unusual behaviors during sleep:

- **Don't wake your child.** This can extend the episode. If the child is having a sleep terror, make them feel secure, and it will pass. If they are sleepwalking, guide them back to bed.
- **If your child sleepwalks, lock the doors and windows.** Get an alarm or rig a bell to ring if your child opens their bedroom door. Make sure the path to your room is clutter-free each night.
- **Don't let your child sleep on a top bunk.** If necessary, put the mattress on the floor.
- **In the morning, don't talk about the episode.** This may create fear or anxiety about going to sleep.
- **Enforce healthy sleep habits.** This includes keeping your child on a regular schedule with consistent times for going to bed and waking up. Also, make sure your child is getting enough sleep.

Unusual behaviors during sleep

memory associated with the dream still lingering. With a sleep terror, a child remains asleep during the whole episode, and most children won't remember having a sleep terror.

Confusional arousals and sleep terrors are most common in children between the ages of 1 and 12 years. Typically, a child will outgrow it.

If your child has sleep terrors, mention it to your child's doctor at the next visit. In most cases, no treatment is necessary, unless there are concerns about safety. Contact a doctor if you believe your child is at risk of injury or other symptoms have appeared.

Some adults also experience confusional arousals, though this is rare. The condition can be brought on by sleep deprivation, which may stem from another sleep disorder. Sleep medications also can contribute to confusional arousals. If you're taking a sleep aid and wake up confused and disoriented, let your doctor know.

OTHER BEHAVIORS

Many other behaviors can develop when you don't wake completely after being disturbed while in a deep sleep.

Sleep talking

Some people moan, mumble or make other incomprehensible sounds while sleeping. When these utterances can be understood, it's known as sleep talking (somniloquy). In most cases sleep talking requires no treatment. It may be triggered by certain medications, including sedatives, and changing the medications may bring an end to the vocalizations. In extreme cases a bed partner may have to sleep separately to get a good night's sleep.

Sexsomnia

Unusual sleep behaviors can also include making sexual advances while asleep. Known as sexsomnia, this can include masturbation or fondling and sexual intercourse with a bed partner. These instances happen when a person is in deep sleep, and there's no recollection of the behavior the next morning.

The condition is more common in men than women. In some cases, medication can be helpful. If the episodes are triggered by another sleep disorder, treating that condition can sometimes end the sexual behavior. For example, some people may experience fewer episodes after using a positive airway pressure (PAP) device to treat obstructive sleep apnea.

Strange behaviors during dream sleep
Behaviors such as sleepwalking, sleep eating and night terrors occur during non-REM sleep. There are other disorders that unfold during REM sleep. Because REM sleep is the segment of sleep when you dream the most, these conditions are often related to dreams, especially those that evoke powerfully negative emotions, such as nightmares.

TEETH GRINDING AND SLEEP

Teeth grinding is another common behavior during sleep, though it's typically not considered a parasomnia. Known as bruxism — based on the Greek word for gnashing teeth — it usually happens during the lighter stages of sleep and is typically unrelated to a partial arousal during deep sleep or REM.

About 13% of adults grind their teeth during sleep. Stress can be a contributing factor, as can certain substances or medications, including antidepressants, amphetamines and alcohol. The exact cause of bruxism isn't fully understood, however. Obstructive sleep apnea can trigger bruxism, and your doctor might want to conduct a sleep study to see if that's the underlying cause.

Treatment usually relies on a device made by a dentist to protect your teeth from being slowly worn away during episodes. Treating underlying causes also can reduce or prevent the problem.

Sleep paralysis
Sleep paralysis is a potentially terrifying phenomenon that occurs when you wake up but find yourself unable to move. Your mind might still be generating threatening, nightmarish hallucinations, such as an intruder standing beside your bed, but you feel conscious and awake. This disorder occurs because you aren't waking fully from REM sleep, and paralysis that occurs normally during REM sleep to keep you from acting out your dreams is still doing its job, preventing you from moving.

More than 7% of the population experiences sleep paralysis, according to one estimate. It can occur on its own, though it's also a symptom of narcolepsy, where the borders between sleep and wakefulness break down. Sleep paralysis happens more frequently when people are sleeping on their backs. And it can sometimes be prompted by discontinuing certain antidepressant medications.

While sleep paralysis is frightening, especially at first, many people become somewhat accustomed to the condition and learn to simply wait a short time for the episode to pass. In most cases treatment isn't necessary if there aren't any other symptoms. When a person is reassured that the condition isn't harmful, their fear and anxiety during episodes often diminish.

Rapid eye movement sleep behavior disorder
Normally, your body goes into temporary paralysis (atonia) during REM sleep so that you don't act out your dreams. In some people, this paralysis no longer functions as it should, and you're able to move while dreaming. You may find yourself having dreams that involve a confrontation or an attack, possibly by an animal, compelling you to defend yourself or a loved one. You may thrash, punch and kick, while calling out or moaning. Within a minute or so, the movement usually stops.

This condition, known as rapid eye movement sleep behavior disorder, may produce symptoms that resemble confusional arousal, sleepwalking or night terrors. However, while those conditions appear during non-REM sleep, this condition occurs when you're dreaming during REM sleep. Episodes are more common in the second half of the night, when you spend the most time in REM sleep.

REM sleep behavior disorder is relatively rare but increases in frequency with age, affecting about 2% of older adults. The condition can be brought on by some medications or by degeneration of certain brain cells, and it may also be associated with other medical conditions.

Some cases of REM sleep behavior disorder begin after taking medications affecting serotonin, a brain neurotransmitter that helps regulate sleep and mood, among other things. This can include classes of medications often used to treat depression, such as selective serotonin reuptake inhibitors (SSRIs) and serotonin-norepinephrine reuptake inhibitors (SNRIs). When REM sleep behavior disorder occurs in individuals younger than age 40, medications are often the cause.

The condition also can be an early sign of Parkinson's disease or Lewy body dementia. More than 33% of people with Parkinson's disease and 80% of people with Lewy body dementia also have REM sleep behavior disorder. REM sleep behavior disorder may occur with no features of Parkinson's disease or Lewy body dementia. People with this condition, called isolated REM sleep behavior disorder, may over time be at increased risk of developing Parkinson's disease or Lewy body dementia.

Narcolepsy is associated with the condition as well. About half of people with narcolepsy also have REM sleep behavior disorder. If you've been diagnosed with narcolepsy, your doctor may ask questions to determine whether you sleepwalk.

Diagnosing REM sleep behavior disorder requires a sleep study in a sleep clinic, where video is used to identify physical movement during REM sleep. A bed partner can often add important information about your activity during sleep and may be invited to attend your medical appointment.

Safety should be an immediate concern for someone with this condition, keeping in mind that bed partners are at risk, too. The bedroom should be safe, with nothing sharp or dangerous near the bed. In some cases, alarms on the bed and door may be necessary. In cases where the risk of hurting someone is great, there may be a need to sleep alone.

When antidepressants are the cause, stopping the medications can sometimes resolve the problem. Other medications, including melatonin supplements or the drug clonazepam, may also help manage the condition. But don't stop taking antidepressants or other medications without consulting your doctor.

Nightmare disorder
A nightmare may be just a dream, but it carries real emotional weight that can affect your sleep and waking hours alike. A nightmare can overwhelm your sleeping mind with negative emotions, inducing such potent fear and panic that it wakes you.

Everyone has an occasional nightmare. Some don't necessarily have an identifiable cause or an apparent relation to your waking life. These are sometimes called idiopathic nightmares.

Other nightmares are clearly associated with a specific trauma, with the content of the dream somehow harkening back to a pivotal negative event in your life. These nightmares can become frequent, and they're a common precursor and symptom of post-traumatic stress disorder. Some individuals may be genetically predisposed to having nightmares triggered by trauma.

When nightmares become frequent or last for a while, they can rise to the level of a nightmare disorder, a condition that affects your ability to sleep and your quality of life.

Nightmare disorder is characterized by repeated, extended bad dreams involving a threat to your survival, safety or physical well-being. When you wake up, you quickly become aware that you were dreaming, but the nightmare sticks in your memory. The condition may impair your ability to work and socialize by affecting your mood, your capacity to think and your energy level. You may be sleepy during the day, yet not want to go to bed at night because of anxiety about having a bad dream.

Approximately 4% of adults have nightmare disorder. In some cases, the nightmares might be related to other psychological disorders, including schizophrenia, depression or anxiety.

Treatment for this type of sleep disorder may include imagery rehearsal techniques that teach you how to influence your thinking and even help steer your dreams in a more positive direction. With imagery rehearsal, you reshape the negative content of your dreams while you're awake, essentially writing a more positive script to your dream scenario, which then carries over to your dreams during sleep. Some people also benefit from medication.

TREATING PARASOMNIAS

Treatment for parasomnias varies by condition. Also, if another condition is disturbing your sleep and triggering episodes, the first step is generally to treat that condition. For example, diagnosing and treating obstructive sleep apnea may reduce sleepwalking.

Medication

Sometimes changing your medications can be part of your treatment. One of the most common sleep aids, zolpidem (Ambien), has been associated with sleepwalking and other unusual behaviors during sleep. If you take this medication and have any symptoms of parasomnias, your doctor may want to switch you to a different medication.

Treatment also may include prescribing medication to help treat your parasomnia. Clonazepam (Klonopin) is an anti-seizure drug sometimes used to treat parasomnias. However, not all sleep experts believe the medication is effective for parasomnias. Your doctor might prescribe it to see if it benefits you.

In some cases of sleep-related eating disorder, your doctor may prescribe topiramate (Eprontia, Topamax, others), a medication developed for preventing seizures or migraines. Several small studies suggest that some people taking topiramate have fewer nighttime eating episodes and lose weight. However, some of those studies also indicate that many people discontinue this medication because of its adverse effects.

Prazosin (Minipress), a medication approved to treat high blood pressure, is sometimes prescribed off-label for people who have frequent nightmares associated with post-traumatic stress disorder (PTSD). However, some research suggests this medication may not be effective for everyone. A study sponsored by the U.S. Department of Veterans Affairs concluded that the medication was no more effective than a placebo for helping ease nightmares in a large group of combat veterans.

Hypnosis

Hypnosis may be beneficial to some people who experience unusual behaviors during sleep, such as sleepwalking, sleep talking and frequent nightmares.

Hypnosis used in a clinical setting isn't like what you see in movies or on TV. It involves a heightened sense of concentration achieved through intense relaxation, putting you in a state to be especially focused on a suggestion. You remain conscious during the therapy, and most people have clear memories of the session from beginning to end. After one or two training sessions with a specialist, you can perform hypnosis on your own at home.

In one long-term study, 36 people who frequently experienced nightmares, sleep terrors or sleepwalking were trained in hypnosis by a specialist. After one or two sessions with the specialist, the study participants were free to practice hypnosis on their own at home. Five years later, 40% of the participants said they were still much improved or no longer had symptoms. The best results were found among those being treated for nightmares and sleepwalking.

Clinical hypnosis has also been found to be effective for confusional arousals and sleep-related eating disorders. These behaviors can become almost habitual, and a positive suggestion during hypnosis may help break the habit.

Hypnosis training usually includes three parts. First, you're given a step-by-step guide for achieving intense relaxation. This is followed by a suggestion or instructions to positively affect your behavior. You're then gently reoriented to your environment after the completion of the suggestion. A suggestion for someone who sleepwalks might be based around the idea that the next time they get out of bed they should turn around and get back into bed.

Hypnosis practiced in training sessions is relatively brief and may last just 10 to 15 minutes. The session may be recorded so that you can listen to it at home to learn the techniques.

For people with unwanted sleep-related behaviors who are otherwise mentally healthy, hypnosis is a very low-risk therapy with the potential for benefit. Hypnosis generally isn't well suited, however, for someone with an active mental health condition such as depression or post-traumatic stress disorder.

If you believe hypnosis might help you with a sleep-related disorder, discuss it with your doctor. Some sleep centers have specialists who are trained in hypnosis.

Sleep habits

With many unusual sleep-related behaviors, lifestyle strategies that promote good sleep may help reduce symptoms. Develop a consistent schedule for going to bed at night and waking in the morning. Make your room quiet and dark. Avoid things that can disturb or fragment sleep, such as alcohol, caffeine, and pets or kids in bed.

In children who sleepwalk, some parents have found success with a technique called anticipatory waking. Just prior to when the episode usually takes place, the parents wake the child, then help them get back to sleep, preventing the onset of the behavior.

13

Internal sleep-clock disorders

When your body is working as it should, you feel alert in the morning, but may find yourself becoming a bit sluggish in midafternoon. Later in the day, you perk up again before becoming sleepy as the evening progresses. This daily waxing and waning of sleepiness is a small element of your circadian rhythm, a powerful internal force that relies on light from the sun to keep your body running on a schedule.

Humans are hardwired to live on a planet with a 24-hour day. Deep inside your brain, a tiny bundle of neurons no bigger in size than a seed serves as your body's master clock (see page 22). This densely packed knot of cells, called the suprachiasmatic nucleus, relies on your eyes to send it signals about how light or dark it is outside, thereby keeping your body aligned with night and day, making you sleepy in the evening and alert and awake come morning.

Like any clock, however, the suprachiasmatic nucleus can sometimes have trouble keeping time. When this internal master clock falls out of sync with the sun and the 24-hour day, you may find yourself feeling sleepy throughout the day and alert at night. Your schedule may not match the one you must keep for work or school. At times, sleep may become unattainable, even though you're exhausted. Gastrointestinal distress, concentration problems and lack of energy (lethargy) may develop. You may also feel moody and irritable, possibly leading to friction in personal relationships or at work.

Several things can cause your master clock to stray from its standard 24-hour cycle. Some are the result of attempts to defy the circadian rhythms your body would naturally follow, such as working late shifts or flying across multiple time zones. Other circadian rhythm disorders are driven by internal causes, including aging, genetics or a medical condition such as dementia, blindness or a brain injury.

RECOGNIZED DISORDERS

There are six recognized circadian rhythm disorders, each with a different cause and often different symptoms.

Shift work disorder
An increasing number of people work outside the standard 9 a.m. to 5 p.m. workday, with about 15% to 20% of U.S. workers on the job during the evening or overnight, on shift work. Shift work can be hard on your body, which is constantly straining against all the signals it receives to sleep at night and to be awake during the day.

This constant tension can lead to what's called shift work disorder, in which you don't get the sleep you need to function well. Insomnia may keep you awake when you're home, and fatigue or sleepiness may prevent you from performing your best at work. About 1 in 3 people who work nights develop shift work disorder.

Shift work is associated with several negative health outcomes, including an increased risk of cardiovascular disease and some cancers. Weight gain is common, and there's an increased risk of glucose intolerance, which can lead to type 2 diabetes. Shift workers are also prone to more mental health problems, including depression and anxiety.

Managing the disorder
To help reduce the negative health effects of shift work, some people nap before heading to work. You might find that you need two sessions of sleep, one after work and another after a meal. This may also help you perform better on the job.

It's a good idea to be aware of light exposure, too. A workplace with bright lights can help you remain alert. If you're having difficulty staying awake and attentive, your doctor might prescribe medications to help you maintain alertness during your evening or night shifts.

After your shift, preventing bright light from shining into your eyes, perhaps by wearing sunglasses, will help your body prepare for sleep. Your bedroom should be as dark and quiet as possible. Also make sure to turn off your phone to avoid interruptions.

If possible, it's best to keep to the same sleep schedule on your days off rather than switch to the standard sleep routine that your friends and family are on.

Later in this chapter, we discuss how melatonin at bedtime may also help you maintain a nontraditional sleep schedule.

Jet lag disorder

Anyone who travels long distances by plane has probably experienced jet lag — you're in one time zone, but your body thinks it's in another. You find yourself feeling awake when you want to be asleep and sleepy when you'd like to be awake. Unlike your mobile phone, your internal clock doesn't reset instantly to local time when your plane touches down. It needs a few days to become aligned with the new time zone. Symptoms of jet lag typically appear when you fly across at least two time zones, and they tend to be worse when you travel east versus west.

While jet lag can be a drag on your performance and energy level, it's relatively short-lived and usually isn't a serious long-term health concern. As a rule of thumb, most people will recover on their own at the rate of one time zone, or one hour, per day.

To help lessen jet lag, it's best to avoid alcohol when flying. Also, if you're traveling for business, try to schedule important meetings as close as possible to a time when you're likely to be awake and alert back home.

Well-timed use of melatonin and awareness of how exposure to light might be affecting your circadian rhythms can help minimize jet lag, as explained later in this chapter.

Delayed sleep-wake phase disorder
With delayed sleep-wake phase disorder, your body clock always lags behind normal circadian rhythms, and you only feel like falling asleep late in the night or early in the morning. Because the rest of the world operates within a time frame different from your biological clock, you're compelled to wake in the middle of your body's preferred sleep time and forced to try to sleep before your body is ready. This makes it hard to fall asleep and wake up.

One of the most common circadian rhythm disorders, this condition often leads to a lack of sleep and daytime fatigue. It may also lead to certain psychiatric conditions, including anxiety and depression.

Delayed sleep-wake phase disorder occurs most frequently in teenagers and young adults. While it's normal for teenagers to become night owls, with this condition symptoms are generally more severe, causing disruptions to daily life, such as missing school or work.

To be diagnosed with the disorder, your sleep patterns must be at least two hours delayed from standard patterns, though the delay can be as much as six hours. You may be unable to sleep before, say, 3 a.m., find it difficult to wake for school or work, and be drowsy during the daytime, especially in the morning. Without an alarm and obligations, you would likely sleep until 10 or 11 a.m. Often a person with the disorder will get a full night's sleep at their preferred time, if allowed to do so.

Treatment may involve well-timed melatonin and light therapy to reset your internal clock. Whatever your age, reducing exposure to light and screens in the evening can help prepare your body for sleep by encouraging the natural release of melatonin.

Advanced sleep-wake phase disorder
In this disorder, your body clock is working ahead of standard circadian rhythms. You may find yourself waking up earlier in the morning and feeling sleepy earlier in the evening than you'd like.

Individuals with this condition typically have sleep schedules that are at least three hours earlier than standard rhythms. For example, you may fall asleep at 6 p.m. and wake at 2 a.m. Your sleep quality may be good, but it's occurring earlier than you want it to.

This disorder is most commonly found among older adults and the elderly. Researchers have found a genetic link to advanced sleep-wake phase disorder that may contribute to the condition when it appears in younger people.

Some people can adapt to the condition and may not need treatment. For others, it can lead to sleep deprivation and isolation. It can be difficult to socialize at night, and family life and work may suffer. If you drive, you risk falling asleep behind the wheel in the evening or at night.

For severe cases, treatment with light therapy and melatonin can help lessen symptoms. The timing of these treatments is discussed later in this chapter.

Non-24-hour sleep-wake rhythm disorder
Some people fall out of sync with the standard 24-hour day and their sleep-wake cycle grows incrementally longer by about 20 minutes each day. They get sleepy and wake up a little later each day. Eventually, people with the disorder may find themselves getting their primary session of sleep in the middle of the afternoon instead of at night.

Most people have a circadian rhythm that's prone to run slightly longer than 24 hours. However, daily exposure to light resets your internal clock to keep your body on a 24-hour cycle. With non-24-hour sleep-wake rhythm disorder, the clock doesn't get reset, allowing people's daily physiological schedule to shift later each day. This condition is considered rare, occurring in fewer than 1 in 2,000 people. However, it's common in people who are completely blind and unable to receive light signals that keep their circadian rhythms aligned with the 24-hour day.

Treatment typically includes melatonin or prescription medications that mimic melatonin to keep the body on a 24-hour schedule.

Irregular sleep-wake rhythm disorder
With this disorder, the body's internal clock has lost its ability to keep time. Sleep and wakefulness no longer fall into their divisions of night

and day, and they generally alternate around the clock. Your nighttime sleep is interrupted because you feel awake, and you nap during the day to relieve sleepiness. In addition, you may not feel rested after sleep.

Individuals with this disorder often have several short periods of sleep in a 24-hour day, and it may not be clear which of these is their primary sleep time. Instead, sleep resembles a succession of naps, much like the pattern of a newborn.

Irregular sleep-wake rhythm disorder is usually associated with neurological disorders such as brain damage or dementia, and it isn't uncommon in memory care units of skilled nursing facilities.

Treatment may include melatonin supplements as well as scheduling daily activities that are stimulating.

WHEN TO SEE A DOCTOR

A medical professional can determine whether you have a circadian rhythm disorder by learning about your sleep schedule and your symptoms, and in some cases, running some tests.

You may be asked detailed questions about your sleep patterns — including when you go to bed, when you fall asleep and when you wake up — as well as whether you feel drowsy or fatigued during the day. You also may be asked to fill out a sleep log for 1 to 2 weeks, where you will compile a detailed account of when and how much you sleep. Questionnaires designed to determine "morningness" or "eveningness" can help reveal whether your circadian rhythms are advanced, delayed or normal (see page 49).

Tests used in diagnosing circadian rhythm disorders vary depending on symptoms. Actigraphy, which measures motion with a watch-like device worn on your wrist, is sometimes used to track when you're awake and when you're asleep. An overnight sleep study (polysomnography) isn't required to diagnose a circadian rhythm disorder. However, it may be done to determine if another sleep disorder, such as obstructive sleep apnea, is contributing to your symptoms.

Your doctor will also make sure that your nonstandard sleep schedule isn't an effect of a medication you're taking or another medical condition.

TREATMENT

For many circadian rhythm disorders, your internal clock can be nudged forward or backward with light therapy and melatonin supplements. In mild, temporary cases, such as jet lag disorder, your internal clock will correct itself. For some disorders and in case of more severe symptoms, medications may be helpful.

Often, getting into a regular sleep schedule will bring some improvement to your symptoms and help you feel better. A regular sleep schedule also will allow other treatments to work as effectively as possible.

Lifestyle choices can also help you manage circadian rhythm disorders. They include the following strategies:

- **Make your bed a place for sleep.** Your bedroom shouldn't be a place for work, watching TV or looking at your laptop or phone.
- **Eat meals on a schedule.** Just as with sleep, it's helpful to establish a routine for when you eat. Regular meals are one of the cues your body uses to set its internal clock.
- **Limit naps.** An afternoon nap can interfere with your ability to fall asleep at night. However, if you work at night, you might find an afternoon nap helps you feel better and improves your performance at work.
- **Avoid alcohol and nicotine.** They can interfere with sleep, especially when used near bedtime.

Light therapy

Light is a potent force for resetting your internal body clock. Cues your brain uses to regulate its internal clock are called zeitgebers, and light is the most powerful one of all. Being conscious of when you're exposed to light during your day can help you stay on a standard circadian rhythm.

If you're not getting enough light or not getting light at the right time of day, your doctor may prescribe a light box to help reset your circadian rhythm. This is a device that looks something like a TV or a computer monitor and delivers bright, therapeutic light. Light boxes typically have a light intensity of 10,000 lux and emit a broad light spectrum similar to sunlight.

The recommended distance when using a light therapy device is usually between 16 and 24 inches from your face, with the light indirectly pointing toward your eyes. Angling the light correctly is important to mimic the natural path of sunlight and to stimulate the appropriate photoreceptors in the eyes. It's generally recommended you use the device every day. Some people use a light box while eating, reading or working, while others just relax during the therapy.

How long and when to use light therapy varies depending on individual needs and the specific disorder being treated. Typically, exposure is around 20 minutes, but it could be longer depending upon the problem being addressed. The timing of light therapy is critical for its effectiveness in shifting the circadian rhythm in the desired direction. Typically, exposure to bright light before sleep pushes your internal clock to a later time, while receiving light after waking pulls the clock to an earlier time. It's important to work with your doctor to make sure you have the timing and length of therapy right.

Light boxes are also available without a prescription. However, be careful which one you buy because many fail to deliver sufficient light intensity.

Melatonin

Your body produces the hormone melatonin to help you sleep. Exposure to light throughout the day is the primary signal your body relies upon to increase melatonin in the evening. If your circadian rhythms are disrupted, your body may not produce enough melatonin at the right time, and taking a melatonin supplement may help you develop and keep to the sleep schedule you want.

Melatonin is sold over the counter in pharmacies or grocery stores and is commonly used to help establish a healthy circadian rhythm. When melatonin is taken to help set your body clock, your doctor may recommend a very low dose of 1 milligram (mg). This is well below the dose manufacturers often recommend when the hormone is used as a sleep aid, which can be as high as 10 mg or more. Dosages of 10 mg or more are much higher than natural levels of the hormone.

Higher levels of melatonin may be effective in helping to promote sleep and treating certain sleep disorders, but they don't necessarily lead to better sleep quality or longer sleep duration for everyone.

Your body's response to the hormone can vary based on individual sensitivity, the timing of when it's taken and the reason you're taking it.

Melatonin isn't a medicine, and it's regulated as a supplement by the Food and Drug Administration (FDA). Because the regulation of supplements isn't as strict as for medications, melatonin supplements can be contaminated with impurities and the dosage can vary widely from what the label says. Purchase melatonin only from reputable supplement manufacturers and look for a seal of approval from one of two nongovernmental quality monitors, United States Pharmacopeia (USP) or NSF International.

WHAT TO LOOK FOR IN A LIGHT BOX

For light therapy to be effective and safe, it's important to purchase a device with the right technical specifications. Here are some key specifications to consider:

1. **Light intensity.** The intensity of light is measured in lux, and for therapeutic purposes, a brightness of about 10,000 lux is typically recommended to mimic the intensity of sunlight after sunrise or before sunset. This level of intensity is considered effective for resetting the body's circadian rhythm when used appropriately.
2. **Light spectrum.** The most effective light therapy lamps emit a broad spectrum of light, with some focusing on blue light wavelengths (around 460 nanometers) that are particularly influential in regulating the circadian rhythm. Clinical tests aren't conclusive regarding the importance of specific wavelengths. Some devices offer options to filter out UV light to protect the skin and eyes.
3. **Flicker.** High-quality light therapy devices should minimize flicker to reduce eyestrain and discomfort during use. LED-based devices often offer the most stable light output.

Coordinating light exposure and melatonin

Treatment for circadian rhythm disorders often includes a combination of low doses of melatonin supplements and high exposure to light. Timing is everything and varies by condition. It's important to understand how these two treatments, light and melatonin, can work together to reset your internal clock.

Light helps keep your internal clock running on time. Your eyes not only are wired to the parts of your brain responsible for vision but also connect to the hypothalamus and your body's master clock.

Experiments performed decades ago revealed that when people are kept in pitch-blackness their circadian rhythms fall out of sync and

4. **Safety and certification.** Light therapy devices should be tested for safety and efficacy, ideally holding certification from recognized standards organizations. To avoid harm, it's important to ensure that the device emits negligible amounts of UV light.
5. **Adjustability.** Some light therapy devices come with features such as adjustable brightness, timers and even sunrise simulation to gently wake the user. These features can enhance their effectiveness and user experience.

When choosing a light therapy device, consider these specifications in conjunction with your individual needs and preferences. Consulting with a healthcare professional experienced in sleep medicine can help determine the most appropriate device and regimen. For individuals with certain eye conditions or those taking medications that increase photosensitivity, special considerations may be necessary to ensure safety during light therapy.

begin shifting. When humans live without light, their bodies migrate from a 24-hour day to a day that's longer than 24 hours. The research established that light is primarily responsible for resetting your internal clock every day and for keeping your circadian rhythms on a 24-hour timetable. (It also shows why adolescents who spend too much time in the basement playing video games can slip into an irregular, unhealthy sleep schedule.)

Melatonin is one of the key hormones in your body's signaling system that brings on sleep and maintains it through the night. A rise in melatonin levels is a signal to your entire body that biological night is coming.

Together, these two potent signaling systems — melatonin and light — can be used to get your body's internal clock and your circadian rhythms more aligned with what's standard. Among medical experts, this coordinated approach is often referred to as the phase response curve. Importantly, the timing of each of the treatments will determine the direction in which your internal clock moves, like deciding whether to set your watch ahead or back.

- **If you fall asleep too late.** With delayed sleep-wake phase disorder, you need to move your internal clock earlier. To do this, treatment typically consists of exposure to bright light early in the morning, minimizing light late in the day and a low dose of melatonin before a standard bedtime.
- **If you're going to bed and waking too early.** With advanced sleep-wake phase disorder, you want to take low-dose melatonin in the morning and avoid bright light early in the day. Exposure to bright light late in the day will hold off sleepiness and nudge your bedtime to later at night, which is the goal. As your sleep pattern shifts, the timing of these two therapies may require adjustment.
- **For non-24-hour circadian rhythm disorder.** Because this condition is most common in people who are blind, melatonin is the primary treatment and light treatment typically isn't used. Treatment may also involve other factors that have some influence on your body clock, such as when you eat meals.
- **For jet lag.** Exposure to bright light before sleep sets your internal clock later and can be helpful for someone traveling across multiple time zones from east to west. Exposure to bright light after

waking up helps someone who's traveling thousands of miles from west to east. Doing the opposite of this can worsen jet lag symptoms.

Melatonin has been shown to help some people adjust to a new time zone and reduce symptoms of jet lag. When you travel east, take melatonin before bed at your destination for several days. If you fly west, take melatonin in the morning. Alternatively, you can take melatonin about 30 minutes before you want to sleep.

- **If you work evening or night shifts.** A session of bright light therapy before work can help you feel more alert. A bright workplace will also help keep your circadian rhythm operating during nontraditional hours. After work, wear sunglasses on the way home to minimize light exposure to your eyes — you don't want to alert your brain to the fact that it's morning. Taking melatonin at your bedtime may help keep your circadian rhythm in line with your night work schedule.

Given its complexity, along with individual variability in circadian rhythms, the coordination of light therapy and melatonin should be done in consultation with your doctor or a sleep specialist. A personalized approach increases the chances of success.

Medications and other substances

Medications also can play a role in treating some circadian rhythm disorders.

Melatonin receptor agonists
Some medicines imitate melatonin so closely that the brain's signaling system accepts them as the real thing. Tasimelteon (Hetlioz) works on the same receptors that melatonin does and has been approved for treating non-24-hour sleep-wake disorder.

Sleeping pills
Some people rely on prescription sleep aids to manage the symptoms of jet lag or shift work disorder. They include non-benzodiazepine receptor agonists, such as zolpidem (Ambien) or eszopiclone (Lunesta). Because these medications are associated with unusual behaviors in

some people, it's best not to take them for the first time when you are away from home.

Wakefulness-promoting medications
These include the drugs modafinil (Provigil) and armodafinil (Nuvigil). Wakefulness-promoting agents are used to treat the sleepiness that comes with circadian rhythm disorders. Because of the way they work, the medications can help you feel alert when you need to be. Unlike many other stimulants, their effects typically last a short time, making them less likely to interfere with sleep. Some people with shift work disorder benefit from these medications.

Caffeine
Caffeine is a stimulant that can be used in moderation to help people reduce sleepiness. If you're a shift worker, a cup of coffee early in your day may help you wake up and feel sharp. Caffeine can also be helpful when managing jet lag. However, caffeine within 6 to 8 hours of your bedtime can prevent you from getting a good night's sleep.

14

Medical conditions and medications

Poor sleep is often related to a separate medical condition that makes it difficult to get a good night's rest. It might be chronic pain from a musculoskeletal disorder, such as arthritis, or breathing difficulties associated with chronic obstructive pulmonary disease (COPD) or another lung condition. When you don't feel well, sleep may not come easily.

Other medical conditions that can interfere with sleep include heartburn, cardiovascular disease, diabetes, kidney disease, thyroid disease and neurological disorders. The stress of illness, especially chronic illness, can lead to insomnia and daytime drowsiness. In addition, some medications you take to treat an illness can make it more difficult for you to sleep at night.

If you're having trouble sleeping and you have a medical condition, talk to your doctor. It's important to find out if your illness may be contributing to your sleep woes, and if there are changes you might make to your treatment plan to improve your sleep.

In this chapter, we discuss a few specific illnesses — infection, cancer and dementia — and their impact on sleep. We also review some commonly used medications that can interfere with sleep.

INFECTION

It's becoming increasingly clear that sleep and the body's immune system are closely related. Consistent sleep strengthens your immune system, helping to prevent illness. Lack of sleep, on the other hand, can throw it off. Evidence indicates that both short- and long-term sleep deprivation can make you sick. When you're tired, even from just one night of poor sleep, brain regulation of the immune system weakens, making you more susceptible to infections.

The relationship between sleep and your immune system is a two-way street. Activation of the immune system by an infection can disturb sleep, but it can also make you sleep longer and deeper, allowing your body to conserve energy for recovery and focus on fighting the foreign bodies making you sick.

You also sleep a bit differently when fighting an infection. You spend more time in deep sleep and less time in rapid eye movement (REM) sleep. Your body devotes maximum energy to battling the foreign invader making you ill during the deep sleep stage, when your immune system is most active.

Sleep on it

Early in an infection, your body activates an inflammatory response that typically prompts a fever and also makes you feel tired and want to sleep. Often, it's easy to fall asleep when you're ill.

Sometimes, though, being sick can make it more difficult to sleep. Some people find it difficult to fall asleep when they have a fever, even though they feel extremely tired. A common cold, caused by a viral infection, can sometimes lead to mild short-term insomnia.

When you become ill, listen to your body's pleas to get more sleep. Sleeping will help you get better faster. If you can't sleep, stay in bed and rest. Once you've recovered, it's important to resume good sleep habits and get back to a consistent sleep schedule.

The COVID-19 pandemic that emerged in 2020 had a great impact on sleep for millions of people. Individuals with acute COVID infection often slept for long periods. Some people continue to have ongoing symptoms of COVID infection, a condition called long COVID. About 40% of individuals with long COVID report having sleep difficulties, including insomnia, waking up in the night, daytime sleepiness and not feeling refreshed in the morning.

Cases of insomnia also increased during the peak of the pandemic, largely because of the disease's disruption to daily life.

If you're struggling to sleep, whether or not you think there's a COVID tie-in, consult your doctor or a sleep specialist. Also consider lifestyle changes to improve your sleep, as discussed in Chapter 4.

CANCER

A diagnosis of cancer can affect all aspects of your health and life, including how well you sleep and your energy levels during the day. More than half of people with cancer experience sleep problems, a much higher percentage than the general population. Sleep difficulties can begin even before diagnosis, last through treatment and continue for many years into the future. Difficulty sleeping often ranks high on the list of how cancer adversely impacts daily life.

Addressing sleep problems is an important part of treating cancer. During treatment, you need sleep to stay physically and mentally healthy. Sleep powers up your immune system, gives your body time to repair cells and tissues, and helps you stay emotionally resilient. It maintains your memory, keeps you mentally sharp and enables you to follow sometimes detailed instructions associated with treatment. Studies also suggest that people with cancer who get quality sleep live longer.

But cancer can work against all this, disrupting sleep in several ways and leading to insomnia and an irregular sleep schedule. Sleep problems may be caused by the cancer itself. Pain is common with cancer, which can also make sleep difficult. A tumor may put pressure on parts of your body, making you uncomfortable. And gastrointestinal problems can develop with some cancers, disturbing you at night.

A lot going on

Your body's immune response to cancer can disrupt sleep as well. Cancer activates inflammation, a complex process that produces chemical byproducts that may keep you awake. Tumors also can produce proteins that tend to reduce REM sleep.

In addition, cancer brings mental health challenges that affect sleep, including stress, anxiety and depression. It can be difficult to sleep when you're deeply worried and frightened about your health and family.

Treatment can contribute to sleep difficulties. Surgery, radiation therapy, hormone therapy and medications all can affect sleep, perhaps leaving you tired during the day and awake in the night. During hospital stays, it can be especially difficult to sleep.

Nearly every person with cancer battles against constantly feeling tired. Fatigue can be a distressing side effect of many cancer treatments, including radiation, chemotherapy and immunotherapy and targeted therapies. Unlike when you're simply tired, deep fatigue often isn't alleviated by rest. It can be so severe that it becomes impossible to do most daily activities. Studies suggest that being as active as possible and exercising can help reduce cancer-related fatigue.

Insomnia can persist after cancer treatment is complete. One recent study found more than half of cancer survivors frequently had trouble falling asleep nine years after they were first diagnosed, and more than 1 in 4 were using sleep medications. Breast cancer survivors were the most likely to have sleep problems.

A number of factors can contribute to long-term sleep difficulties, including fear of the cancer recurring, physical pain and anxiety. Cancer also can affect your employment and be a financial drain, causing economic hardship and stress that can interfere with sleep.

It's important to discuss your sleep problems with your doctors. In some cases, you might be referred to a sleep specialist to determine if you have an underlying sleep disorder that also may be hampering your sleep. Before seeing a doctor, you might keep track of your sleep patterns for a couple of weeks, including when you wake in the morning and go to bed at night and details of your sleep routine. This will help your doctor understand exactly what the problem is.

Improving sleep

For individuals with cancer struggling with insomnia, cognitive behavioral therapy for insomnia (CBT-I) often can improve sleep quality and the ability to function during the day. Evidence suggests CBT-I is more effective for improving sleep than sleep medications are.

CBT-I addresses poor sleep habits and helps you control the anxiety and fear that can interfere with sleep. Some of the therapy's

---

YOGA FOR BETTER SLEEP

Yoga is a popular mind-body practice known for promoting relaxation, reducing stress and anxiety, and improving flexibility and strength. It also has been shown to improve sleep. Yoga is sometimes recommended for individuals being treated for cancer to improve their sleep quality. Studies have shown it can be particularly helpful for individuals bothered by stress, anxiety and the physical effects of treatment.

Gentle yoga practices that have been shown to improve sleep include postures (asanas), breath control (pranayama) and meditation. These practices promote relaxation and reduce sympathetic nervous system activity thought to enhance overall sleep quality.

Studies that looked specifically at breast cancer survivors found that regularly practicing yoga can significantly improve sleep quality and reduce the use of sleep medications. This is particularly relevant because sleep issues can persist long after treatment has ended, affecting quality of life and overall well-being.

Another benefit of yoga is that it empowers you to take an active role in your own care and recovery. It's important to note, however, that yoga should complement conventional cancer treatments, not replace them. It also should be tailored to your individual physical capabilities and limitations and is best done with an instructor.

components include mindfulness, relaxation techniques and meditation, which also can help lessen fatigue. (See Chapter 6 for more information on CBT-I.)

Good sleep habits are important when you have cancer. Keep to a regular sleep schedule. Create a restful environment in the bedroom that encourages sleep by making the room cool, quiet and dark. Keep your bedroom free of electronic devices, such as TVs and laptops, and don't look at your phone in bed. It's also important to reduce or avoid substances such as coffee, alcohol and nicotine that can disrupt sleep.

Moderate exercise, including regular walking or gentle yoga, is important for several reasons. It can help you sleep better, reduce fatigue and improve your ability to carry on with daily activities.

Sleep medication can be beneficial in some cases but must be balanced against potential side effects that may pose extra risks if you're taking other complex medications to treat your cancer.

If you're a cancer survivor and you have difficulties sleeping, discuss it with your doctor or a sleep specialist.

DEMENTIA

There are many forms of dementia, an umbrella term for conditions that increasingly diminish the ability to think, remember, speak and remain independent. The best-known and most common form of dementia is Alzheimer's disease.

Symptoms commonly associated with dementia are generally the result of physical changes in the brain that also can dramatically alter sleep patterns. Sleep changes brought on by dementia can cause significant challenges for individuals with dementia and their caregivers alike.

Interestingly, sleep may also play a role in who develops dementia. Getting the right amount of high-quality sleep over your lifetime can help keep your brain healthy. Research strongly suggests that poor sleep over many years may contribute to the onset and progression of dementia.

Because this cause-and-effect relationship between sleep and dementia works both ways — poor-quality sleep contributes to the development of dementia, and dementia diminishes the quality of sleep — the relationship is sometimes called bidirectional.

Brain changes

Between 60% and 80% of people with symptoms of dementia have Alzheimer's disease, which appears most frequently in people 65 years and older. The disease affects some 50 million people and is a leading cause of death in the United States.

Alzheimer's disease results from the accumulation of beta-amyloid and tau proteins produced in the brain. Beta-amyloid is a sticky substance and can form into clumps (plaques), interfering with the ability of brain neurons to communicate with one another. Tau blocks the brain's signaling system by forming threads (tangles) inside neurons. Your immune system responds to the beta-amyloid plaques and tau tangles as if they were invaders, resulting in inflammation and damage to brain cells.

One of the first areas of the brain to be affected is a small cluster of cells called the suprachiasmatic nucleus, your body's master clock. This internal clock tells your body when to produce melatonin, a hormone that plays a central role in sleep. With Alzheimer's disease, the body produces less melatonin, leading to a breakdown in the daily rhythms (circadian rhythms) that keep your body in sync with a 24-hour day.

Sleep problems associated with Alzheimer's disease commonly include difficulty falling asleep at night and an inability to get enough sleep. Some people with dementia no longer follow 24-hour patterns, sleeping on and off around the clock — a few hours in the morning and a few hours in the afternoon, and then only a few hours overnight. This fragmented sleep is of poor quality and not restorative. Sleeping at random times around the clock is known as non-24-hour sleep-wake cycle disorder. This is common in dementia.

In addition, dementia can affect normal sleep stages. People with Alzheimer's disease average less time in deep sleep and REM sleep compared to healthy adults. Spending more time in lighter stages of sleep doesn't provide the important restorative functions of deep sleep and REM sleep.

Other forms of dementia include dementia with Lewy bodies and Parkinson's disease with dementia. Sleep problems, especially insomnia and excessive daytime sleepiness, are extremely common in these forms as well, affecting 9 out of 10 people with the conditions.

Individuals with Parkinson's disease and Lewy body dementia commonly experience REM sleep behavior disorder, in which a person acts out their dreams, sometimes violently. The disorder is less common with Alzheimer's disease. Restless legs syndrome may develop with Lewy body dementia or Parkinson's disease.

Treatment
It's especially important to address sleep problems in someone living at home with dementia. Irregular sleep can create significant demands and challenges for caregivers, as there's no overnight downtime, because the person with dementia isn't sleeping through the night. Nighttime wandering is one of the most common reasons that care can no longer be provided at home.

When seeing a doctor, a caregiver is often best able to provide a detailed history of the sleep problems involved, which is important in the development of a treatment plan. Treatment may include lifestyle adjustments, behavioral strategies, medications, light exposure and melatonin.

The first step in determining how best to address sleep problems associated with dementia is to determine if another disorder is contributing to the problem. For example, obstructive sleep apnea is common among people with Alzheimer's disease. Treatment with positive airway pressure (PAP) devices has been shown to improve some of the cognitive symptoms of Alzheimer's disease by increasing oxygen levels in blood and improving sleep.

Treating restless legs syndrome, which frequently develops in people with Lewy body dementia and Parkinson's disease, may include medications or supplements to correct iron deficiency. This can often improve sleep.

Treatment also may include scheduled daytime activities, including physical exercise and social activities, to help individuals stay awake during the day and encourage sleep at night. Because the internal signaling system for when to become sleepy or alert has broken down, activities can provide external cues for when it's time to be awake or to sleep.

Light therapy during the day and a low-light environment at night can be helpful. Bright light therapy in the morning has been shown to help people with dementia fall asleep faster at night, sleep longer and spend less time awake in bed.

Melatonin supplements also may improve sleep. Melatonin levels often are reduced among individuals with Alzheimer's disease, upsetting the body's circadian rhythms. Some studies suggest melatonin supplements taken before bedtime may promote longer sleep during the night.

The medication tasimelteon (Hetlioz) is approved for the treatment of non-24-hour sleep-wake disorder. However, because of the high cost of the drug, doctors may suggest a trial of melatonin supplements first.

Certain hypnotic medications also may be prescribed to improve sleep. However, there's some concern these medications can aggravate other dementia symptoms. For some, the potential benefit of the medication to alleviate sleep problems outweighs the risk it may worsen cognitive symptoms.

MEDICATIONS THAT DISTURB SLEEP

Prescription medications have become a part of everyday life. By one estimate, 66% of U.S. adults take prescription medications. Along with the sometimes life-changing benefits of these medications can come side effects, often involving sleep. In some cases, a medication could be interfering with your ability to get enough quality sleep. (On occasion, a medication to treat an unrelated condition might actually improve your sleep.)

The following are some of the most common medications known to affect sleep.

Blood pressure medications

Drugs taken to lower high blood pressure (hypertension) are some of the most commonly prescribed drugs in use today. The top four types of anti-hypertensive medications alone are taken by more than 60 million people in the United States.

Blood pressure medications may either help or harm your ability to sleep. Some blood pressure medications are beneficial because they can help treat obstructive sleep apnea. High blood pressure and obstructive sleep apnea commonly go hand in hand. Some 30% of individuals with high blood pressure and 80% of those with medication-resistant high blood pressure also have obstructive sleep apnea.

Among these individuals, research shows that treating high blood pressure can reduce the nighttime awakenings characteristic of sleep apnea. Sleep disturbances associated with sleep apnea occur when soft tissues of the upper airway collapse. Some blood pressure medications appear to help stabilize the airway, potentially reducing the number of apnea episodes.

Other blood pressure medications, however, do just the opposite, interfering with sleep:

- **Lisinopril (Zestril).** This medication, known as an ACE inhibitor, relaxes blood vessels and reduces blood pressure by blocking the formation of a chemical that narrows them. Though not common, a known side effect of the medication is trouble sleeping. ACE inhibitor medications also can cause a persistent cough that can make it difficult to sleep.
- **Amlodipine (Norvasc).** Amlodipine works by blocking calcium from entering cells. It, too, can interfere with sleep, although this side effect is not common.
- **Beta-blockers, including metoprolol (Lopressor).** This medication can reduce levels of melatonin, a hormone your body produces to promote sleep. Low levels of melatonin can lead to sleep disturbances, including insomnia and unusual dreams, as well as daytime sleepiness.

Antipsychotic and antidepressant medications

Roughly 1% of the population has schizophrenia, an illness that affects a person's thoughts and feelings, sometimes blurring the line between what's real and what's a hallucination. Many people with schizophrenia also experience sleep disorders, including insomnia, restless legs syndrome and obstructive sleep apnea.

Antipsychotic medications treat schizophrenia. They include the drugs clozapine, olanzapine and quetiapine. Because they're sedatives, antipsychotic medications cause sleepiness. However, they also can increase the risk of weight gain, which can contribute to obstructive sleep apnea.

Antidepressant medications can be both harmful and helpful to sleep. Certain antidepressants can disrupt sleep, including selective serotonin reuptake inhibitors (SSRIs), buprorion and serotonin-norepinephrine reuptake inhibitors (SNRIs). Other antidepressants, however, may improve sleep, including the drugs trazodone and mirtazapine. In fact, trazodone, prescribed in low doses, is now more often used as a sleep aid than it is as an antidepressant.

Because a common symptom of depression is trouble sleeping, it can sometimes be difficult to determine if it's the disease or the medication to treat it that's interfering with sleep. If you believe an antidepressant you're taking may be disrupting your sleep, talk to your doctor. Don't stop taking the drug unless your doctor tells you to.

Erectile dysfunction medications

Many men with obstructive sleep apnea also experience erectile dysfunction. Medication used to treat erectile dysfunction can make sleep apnea worse, however.

The drug sildenafil (Viagra) revolutionized the treatment of erectile dysfunction. However, sildenafil's mechanism of action can lead to muscle relaxation and upper airway congestion, the very things that can contribute to breathing disruption associated with sleep apnea. Using sildenafil is associated with an increase in the number of sleep apnea events and a decrease in levels of oxygen in the blood. Sildenafil also may affect the stages of sleep, increasing time spent in light sleep and decreasing the time in deep sleep.

Others

Other medications guilty of disrupting sleep include:
- Medications that help keep the airways open in the treatment of asthma and chronic obstructive pulmonary disease (COPD), such as theophylline or certain rescue inhalers used in doses higher than typically prescribed.
- Steroid medications, including prednisone or high-dose, high-potency inhaled corticosteroids.

- Medications that contain caffeine or other stimulant ingredients, such as those used to treat attention-deficit/hyperactivity disorder (ADHD) and certain antidepressants.
- Prescription pain medications, which can alter sleep cycles or lead to sleep-disordered breathing.
- Prescription and nonprescription products to curb smoking.

If you believe there may be a link between your sleep problems and the medications you take, talk with your doctor. But don't stop taking any medication on your own. Doing so could cause serious complications to your treatment.

Final thoughts

Now that you've been immersed in the most up-to-date understanding of sleep, what's next? We'd like to leave you with just a few brief, final thoughts about what you can do now.

More than anything, we hope this book has shown you how sleep is connected to every aspect of your health and your overall well-being. The information presented here makes a very compelling case that getting a good night's sleep should be a major priority in your life, just like getting enough exercise and eating a healthy diet. If you don't sleep well, it's time to start fixing that.

You can improve sleep on your own with the relatively straightforward steps outlined in this book, including building a healthy bedtime routine, learning relaxation techniques and being mindful about your use of alcohol and caffeine, among other things.

For remedying some sleep problems, your doctor or a sleep specialist is an essential partner. Modern medicine has developed a wide array of treatments for sleep disorders that can bring life-changing results. Contacting your doctor can be an all-important first step toward better sleep.

And remember, small steps can make a big difference. If you have problems sleeping, don't try to fix everything at once. Start small, and things may well begin to get better, a little bit at a time.

In our years of practice, we've seen countless people improve their sleep, and we've witnessed firsthand how it benefits every aspect of their lives. You can do it, too.

Sleep well!

Additional resources

American Academy of Sleep Medicine
aasm.org/clinical-resources/patient-info/

Centers for Disease Control and Prevention
cdc.gov/sleep/resources/

Circadian Sleep Disorders Network
circadiansleepdisorders.org

KNOW Narcolepsy
knownarcolepsy.com

Mayo Clinic Connect Insomnia & Anxiety Support Group
connect.mayoclinic.org/discussion/insomnia-anxiety/

Mayo Clinic Connect Sleep Health Support Group
connect.mayoclinic.org/group/sleep-health/

Narcolepsy Network
narcolepsynetwork.org

National Sleep Foundation
thensf.org

Project Sleep
project-sleep.com

Restless Legs Syndrome Foundation
rls.org

Sleep Apnea.org
sleepapnea.org

Sleep Foundation
sleepfoundation.org

Wake Up Narcolepsy
wakeupnarcolepsy.org

Index

A

actigraphy, 38–39, 122, 136, 201, 287
adenosine, 60, 61, 87
ADHD, 262, 306
adolescence and teens
    car safety and, 75
    chronotypes in, 49
    circadian rhythm disorders in, 111
    delayed sleep-wake phase disorder in, 111
    school schedules and, 55
    sleep needs in, 44, 45, 50–51
    social jet lag and, 50
    vaping and, 64
advanced sleep-wake phase disorder, 285–286, 292
alarm clocks, 36, 37, 100–102, 113
    snooze features, 68, 100–101
    weekend use, 100–101
alcohol use, 62–63, 87–88, 106–107, 135, 240
    circadian rhythm disorders and, 288
    glymphatic system and, 17
    jet lag and, 284
    restless legs syndrome and, 110, 251, 253
    sleep apnea and, 182, 210
    sleep medications and, 173
    sleep stages and, 41
    sleepwalking and, 270
    snoring and, 192, 193
    teeth grinding and, 275
    time to fall asleep and, 38
Alzheimer's disease, 11, 18, 78, 300–303
    See also dementia
    brain changes in, 301–302
    jet lag and, 50
    treatments for, 302–303
Ambien. *See* zolpidem
American Academy of Sleep Medicine, 39, 43, 46, 123, 151
    on adjusting to daylight saving time, 48
    on cannabis for sleep apnea, 229
    on CBT-I, 137, 140
    on insomnia treatments, 136, 137, 163
    on sleep apnea, 98
    sleep guidelines, 43
    on sleep medications and supplements, 164–165, 168
    on snoring treatments, 193
    on white noise, 98
amygdala, 21, 22, 23, 30
ancient sleep practices, 27
animals, sleep and, 14–15
antidepressants, 157, 162, 163, 172, 242, 250–251, 277–278, 305–306
antihistamines, 163, 164–167, 192, 193

antipsychotics, 251, 270, 304–305
anti-seizure medication, 270, 279
automobile safety. *See* car safety and accidents

B

barriers to sleep, 68–71
   age, 68–69
   menopause, 71
   menstruation, 69–70
   pregnancy, 70–71
basal forebrain, 22, 23
Beck, Aaron, 143
bed partners and bed-sharing, 65–67
   infant bed-sharing cautions, 66
   parasomnias and, 266, 268, 274
   REM sleep behavior disorder and, 277
   sleep apnea and, 66–67, 202, 220
   snoring and, 66–67, 107, 130, 190, 193, 194
bedrooms and sleeping environments, 96–104
   alarm clocks, 100–101
   circadian rhythm disorders and, 288
   clothing, 99
   darkness and light, 97–98
   humidifiers, 193
   insomnia and, 134
   mattresses, 102–103
   parasomnias and, 267, 272, 273, 277
   for people with cancer, 300
   pets in beds, 103–104
   quiet and noise, 98–99
   screens and, 89
   shift work disorder and, 284
   temperature, 99–100
   weighted blankets, 102
benzodiazepines, 156, 160–162, 242, 259
beta-amyloid, 18, 19, 301
beta-blockers, 304
binge eating, 111, 258, 266, 272
biphasic (two-part) sleep, 27
blue-blockers, 58
blue light, 57, 58–59, 89, 97, 290

brain stem, 22, 23, 30, 179, 187
brain waves, 24–25
   alpha, 25, 26
   apnea and, 136, 196–197
   beta, 25
   delta, 25
   gamma, 25
   sleep stages and, 28–29
   testing and monitoring, 40, 41, 118, 136, 196–197, 199, 238
   theta, 25, 26

C

caffeine, 59–62, 134, 300
   in coffee, 59–62, 63, 87–88
   disordered breathing and, 182
   in energy drinks, 59, 60, 62, 88
   interrupted sleep and, 53
   jet lag and, 294
   medications containing, 306
   narcolepsy and, 240
   restless legs syndrome and, 110, 251, 253, 262
   shift workers and, 294
   sleep disorders and, 106–107
   in soda, 60
   stress management and, 65
   in tea, 60, 88, 121
   teens and, 51, 230
   time to fall asleep and, 38
   withdrawal, 88
cancer, 42, 50
   shift work and, 55
   sleep problems due to, 171, 297–300
cannabis, 169–171, 229
cardiovascular health and disease, 77–78, 295
   daylight saving time and, 48
   high blood pressure and, 185
   insomnia and, 74
   Jackson Heart Study, 42
   nicotine and, 88
   poor sleep and, 42, 46, 77–78
   shift work and, 55, 283
   sleep apnea and, 42, 74, 109, 201, 208

car safety and accidents
    cannabis use and, 229
    Epworth Sleepiness Scale and, 117
    narcolepsy and, 232, 238
    poor sleep and, 74, 75
    sleep apnea and, 187, 212
    sleep walking and, 268
CBT-I. *See* cognitive behavioral therapy for insomnia
central sleep apnea, 109, 177, 187, 197, 202–205. *See also* obstructive sleep apnea
    causes of, 202–204
    diagnosing, 204
    treatments for, 204–205
cerebral cortex, 22, 23
    neocortex, 20
    prefrontal cortex, 21, 30
children
    bed-sharing, 65–67
    confusional arousals and sleep terrors in, 272–274
    COVID-19 pandemic and, 55
    exploding head syndrome in, 112
    narcolepsy in, 232
    restless legs syndrome in, 110, 112, 262
    sleep needs in, 43–44
    sleepwalking in, 268, 281
chronotypes, 47, 49, 52, 65
cigarettes. *See* nicotine
circadian rhythm disorders, 110–111, 282–283
    advanced sleep-wake phase disorder, 285–286, 292
    delayed sleep-wake phase disorder, 285, 292
    irregular sleep-wake rhythm disorder, 286–287
    jet lag disorder, 284–285, 288
    lifestyle changes for, 288
    light therapy for, 285, 286, 288–291
    medications for, 293–294
    melatonin for, 285, 286, 287, 288, 289–293
    non-24-hour sleep-wake rhythm disorder, 286, 293, 301
    seeking medical care for, 287
    shift work disorder, 122, 283–284, 293–294
    treatments for, 288–294
circadian rhythms, 13
    appetite and, 86
    cardiovascular health and, 77
    daylight saving time and, 48
    early birds and night owls, 49
    jet lag and, 50
    melatonin and, 58, 69
    REM sleep and, 26
    shift work and, 55
    sleep needs and, 44–50
    sleep regularity and, 41
    suprachiasmatic nucleus and, 23
    zeitgebers, 84, 288
coffee. *See* caffeine
cognitive behavioral therapy (CBT), 143
cognitive behavioral therapy for insomnia (CBT-I), 137–151, 172, 299–300
    apps, 150
    cognitive therapy, 142
    phototherapy, 149
    relaxation therapies, 144–149
    sleep hygiene, 144
    sleep restriction therapy, 140–142, 149–150
    stimulus control therapy, 138–140, 149, 150
cold medications, 251
cold virus, common, 16–17, 296
confusional arousals, 272–274, 276
cortisol, 16, 64, 69, 96, 130
COVID-19 infection, 206, 297
COVID-19 pandemic, 55, 297
COVID-19 vaccine, 17

D

daridorexant, 156, 162
dark environments, 97–98
da Vinci, Leonardo, 13
daylight saving time, 48, 69
deep breathing, 94, 146

delayed sleep-wake phase disorder, 285, 292
dementia, 18, 78–79, 165, 185, 277, 287, 300–303. *See also* Alzheimer's disease
diabetes. *See* type 2 diabetes
dopamine, 110, 248–250, 257–258, 260
dopamine medications, 257–258
doxepin, 163, 164
dreams, 30–34. *See also* nightmares
  ancient views of, 31
  lucid dreams, 33
  sleep cycles and, 31–32
dual orexin receptor antagonists (DORAs), 161–162

E

eating disorders, sleep-related, 11, 265, 270–272, 279, 280
Edison, Thomas, 13
Edluar. *See* zolpidem
EEG, 24, 25, 31, 120, 196–197
Einstein, Albert, 13
electroencephalography (EEG), 24, 25, 31, 120, 196–197
emotions, sleep functions and, 21
energy conservation, 14, 21, 296
energy drinks, 59, 60, 62, 88. *See also* caffeine
eszopiclone, 156, 157–158, 159, 164, 268, 293
exploding head syndrome, 112

F

fish oil, 18
food and diet, sleep and, 86–87
Freud, Sigmund, 31

G

gabapentin, 256, 257
gabapentin enacarbil, 256
gamma-aminobutyric acid (GABA), 23, 62, 155–156, 158–160, 162, 169, 172

gamma-hydroxybutyrate (GHB), 242
gender differences
  barriers to sleep and, 69–71
  insomnia and, 52
  restless legs syndrome and, 52
  sleep apnea and, 52
  sleep needs and, 52
ghrelin, 16, 76, 182
glucose, 17, 76, 186
glucose intolerance, 283
glymphatic system, 17–18, 19, 29
Gralise, 256
growth hormone, 16, 29
guided imagery, 94, 134, 144–146

H

heart attack. *See* cardiovascular health and disease
herbal supplements, 171–172
  jujube seed, 172
  kava, 171–172
  valerian, 165, 171
Horizant, 256
hormones. *See also* melatonin
  cortisol, 16, 64, 69, 96, 130
  ghrelin, 16, 76, 182
  growth hormone, 16, 29
  leptin, 16, 76, 181, 182
  menstruation and, 69
  restless legs syndrome and, 260
  thyroid-stimulating hormone, 16
hypocretin (orexin), 23, 156, 160–162, 235, 236–237, 240, 244
hypothalamus, 22
  damage to, 237
  effect of blue light on, 59
  narcolepsy and, 237
  retinohypothalamic pathway, 57
  role in, 23, 47
  stress and, 64

I

idiopathic insomnia, 242–244. *See also* narcolepsy
immune system, 12, 16–17, 29, 73, 85, 236, 296, 297, 298, 301

infection, 296–297
influenza
    narcolepsy and, 236
    vaccine, 17
insomnia, 123–127
    acute vs. chronic, 127
    causes of, 129–132
    CBT-I, 137–151, 172, 299–300
    depression and, 130
    diagnosing, 128, 134–136
    fatal insomnia, 133
    medications and, 126, 151–152
    risks and costs of, 129
    risks for, 130–131
    seeking medical care for, 132–134
    sleep-wake balance and, 131–132
    symptoms of, 108–109
    three Ps model of, 130–131
    treatments for, 136–152
internal sleep-clock disorders. *See* circadian rhythm disorders
irregular sleep-wake rhythm disorder, 286–287

J

jet lag, 111, 284–285. *See also* social jet lag
    age and, 69
    blue-blockers and, 58
    caffeine and, 294
    light therapy and, 292–293
    melatonin and, 167, 169
jet lag disorder, 284–285, 288

K

kaizen, 83
K-complexes, 25, 28

L

lemborexant, 156, 162
leptin, 16, 76, 181, 182
light therapy, 285, 286, 288–291, 303
Lopressor, 304
lucid dreams, 33

Lunesta, 156, 157–158, 159, 164, 268, 293
Lyrica, 256

M

Maurer, Robert, 83
medications, 154–157. *See also* herbal supplements; melatonin; sleep medications, prescription
    American Academy of Sleep Medicine recommendations, 164–165
    antidepressants, 157, 162, 163, 172, 242, 250–251, 277–278, 305–306
    antihistamine products, 163, 164–167, 192, 193
    antipsychotics, 251, 270, 304–305
    anti-seizure medications, 270, 279
    benzodiazepines, 156, 160–162, 242, 259
    blood pressure medications, 303–304
    cannabis, 169–171, 229
    dopamine medications, 258
    doxepin, 163, 164
    dual orexin receptor antagonists (DORAs), 161–162
    erectile dysfunction medications, 305
    gabapentin, 256, 257
    gamma-aminobutyric acid (GABA), 23, 62, 155–156, 158–160, 162, 169, 172
    history of sleep medications, 155–157
    for idiopathic hypersomnia, 243–244
    for narcolepsy, 241–242
    opioids and, 160, 161, 173
    over-the-counter sleep aids, 163–172
    for parasomnias, 279
    proper use of, 153–154, 172–174
    for restless legs syndrome, 254–259
    semaglutide, 209
    sleep disturbance from, 303–306

Index   315

medications *(continued)*
    for sleep-related eating disorders, 279
    topiramate, 279
meditation, 93–94, 144–145, 299
medulla, 22, 23. *See also* brain stem
melatonin, 16, 47, 167–169
    blue light and, 58
    dementia and, 301, 302, 303, 304
    internal sleep-clock disorders and, 285, 286, 287, 288, 289–293
    jet lag and, 169
    production of, 57
    regulation and labeling of, 168
    REM sleep behavior disorder and, 277–278
memory
    caffeine and, 43, 59
    naps and, 92
    sleep and, 18–21, 65, 73, 297
menopause and perimenopause, 52, 71, 124, 184
metoprolol, 304
midbrain, 22, 23
migration, animal, 15
mnemonic induction of lucid dreams (MILD), 33
muscle relaxation, 148

N

naps, 90–93
    circadian rhythm disorders and, 284, 287, 288
    cultural differences, 86
    insomnia and, 131, 139, 140
    long naps, 91–92, 93
    narcolepsy and, 230, 235, 239, 240, 242–243
    power naps, 91
    pregnancy and, 71
    sleep apnea and, 230, 235, 239, 240, 242–243
    sleep needs by age, 44
    sleep restriction therapy and, 141, 142
    workplace strategies and, 56
narcolepsy, 230–233. *See also* idiopathic insomnia
    diagnosing, 237–240
    driving with, 238–239
    lifestyle changes for, 240–241
    managing, 240–242
    medications for, 241–242
    secondary narcolepsy, 237
    symptoms of, 110, 233–236
    types of, 236–237, 240, 244
Neurontin, 256
nicotine, 63–64, 88–89, 113
    circadian rhythm disorders and, 288
    insomnia and, 134
    narcolepsy and, 241
    restless legs syndrome and, 110, 251
nightmare disorder, 278–279
nightmares, 32, 33, 266, 273, 275, 278–279, 280
non-24-hour sleep-wake rhythm disorder, 286, 293, 301

O

obesity
    poor sleep and, 74–75, 129
    sleep apnea and, 177, 182, 183, 184, 186, 190, 194, 209–210, 224
    social jet lag and, 50
obesity hypoventilation syndrome, 183
obstructive sleep apnea, 175–178. *See also* central sleep apnea
    accidents and, 187
    apnea-hypopnea index (AHI) score, 200
    appetite and, 182
    cannabis and, 229
    causes of and risks factors for, 181–184
    dangers of, 184–189
    daytime sleepiness and, 188
    death and, 189
    deviated septum surgery for, 227
    diabetes and, 186, 190
    diagnosing, 193–202
    excess weight or obesity and, 177, 181, 182, 183, 184, 186, 190, 194, 209–210, 224
    gender differences, 183–184

health and, 183
high blood pressure and, 185–186
home tests, 119–122, 195, 198–202
insomnia and, 188
large neck size and, 190
lifestyle and, 182
mechanics of, 178–181
nighttime urination and, 188–189
normal vs. obstructed breathing, 180
obesity hypoventilation syndrome and, 183
oral anatomy and, 182
oral appliances for, 222–223
positional therapy for, 227–228
positive airway pressure treatments, 210–221
seeking medical care for, 189–193
snoring and, 190–194
statistics, 177
stroke and, 186–187
surgery for, 223–227
symptoms of, 109, 190–191
treatments for, 109–229
weight loss for, 209–210

older adults
advanced sleep-wake phase disorder and, 286
insomnia in, 150
napping and, 93
REM sleep behavior disorder in, 277
sleep medications and, 172
sleep needs in, 45, 52

omega-3 fatty acids, 18
opioids, 160, 161, 173, 195, 203, 242, 259
orexin. See hypocretin
Ozempic, 209

P

parasomnias, 111–112, 264–266
confusional arousals, 272–274, 276
disorders of arousal, 267
hypnosis for, 280–281
lifestyle changes for, 281
medications for, 279
nightmare disorder, 278–279
REM sleep behavior disorder, 196, 276–278, 302
sexsomnia, 274–275
sleep paralysis, 276
sleep-related eating disorder, 270–272
sleep talking, 274, 280
sleep terrors, 112, 268, 272–274, 280
sleepwalking, 29, 111, 181, 196, 265–266, 267–270, 273, 279–280
strange behaviors during dream sleep, 275–279
treatments for, 279–281

Pavlov, Ivan Petrovich, 138–139
perimenopause. See menopause and perimenopause
pets, 103–104
pineal gland, 22, 23, 57, 167
polysomnography. See sleep studies
pons, 22, 23. See also brain stem
poor sleep, consequences of, 72–73, 74–79. See also sleep deprivation and sleep debt
cardiovascular problems, 77–78
dementia, 78–79
obesity, 75–76
performance and safety, 74–75
type 2 diabetes, 76–77

post-traumatic stress disorder, 278–280
pregabalin, 256
pregnancy
barriers to sleep during, 70–71, 124
iron deficiency during, 249
medications during, 172, 241, 255
restless legs syndrome during, 255, 260–261

procrastination, bedtime, 54
progressive muscle relaxation, 94, 147, 148

Q

quiet environments, 98–99

R

ramelteon, 162, 164
rapid eye movement (REM), 25–26, 28, 29–30, 52, 62. See also sleep stages
    bed partners and, 65
    benzodiazepines and, 160
    infection and, 296
    memory system and, 20
    narcolepsy and, 233, 235
    nicotine and, 63
    noise and, 98
    parasomnias and, 266–267, 275–279
    sleep apnea and, 179
rapid eye movement sleep behavior disorder, 196, 276–278, 302
relaxation techniques, 93–95
relaxed breathing exercise, 147
REM. See rapid eye movement
restless legs syndrome, 245–248
    ADHD and, 262
    causes of, 248–251
    children with, 262
    coping with and support for, 261–263
    devices for, 259–261
    diagnosing, 251–252
    dopamine and, 248–249, 258
    genetics and, 249–250
    iron deficiency and, 249
    iron therapy for, 255–256
    lifestyle changes for, 253–254
    massage for, 253
    medications for, 254–259
    pregnancy and, 260–261
    symptoms of, 110, 247–248
    treatments for, 252–261
retinohypothalamic pathway, 57
Rybelsus, 209

S

Schedule I drugs, 170
screens and screen time, 53, 57–59, 134, 139, 285
    blue light from, 57, 58–59, 89, 97, 290
    COVID-19 pandemic and, 55
    teens and, 51

semaglutide, 209
sexsomnia, 274–275
sexual activity, 96
shift work
    caffeine and, 294
    gender differences and, 69
    health risks of, 55, 56, 111, 122, 283, 293–294
    long naps and, 93
    pregnancy and, 70
    sleep health guidelines, 56
short-sleepers, 36
sleep apnea. See central sleep apnea; obstructive sleep apnea
sleep centers, 123
sleep cycles. See sleep stages
sleep deprivation and sleep debt
    biphasic sleep theory and, 27
    consequences of, 73, 74, 79–80, 187–188
    daylight saving time and, 48
    glymphatic system and, 18
    insomnia and, 125, 129
    learning and, 20
    normalization of, 54
    parasomnias and, 267, 269, 270, 274, 286
    paying off sleep debt, 79–80
    signs of, 100
    sleep apnea and, 187–188
    in teens, 51
    vaccination efficacy and, 17
sleep diaries, 118
sleep disorders, 105–106. See also central sleep apnea; circadian rhythm disorders; insomnia; narcolepsy; obstructive sleep apnea; parasomnias; restless legs syndrome
    common disorders, 108–112
    diagnosing, 113–122
    seeking medical care for, 112–113
    warning signs of, 106–108
sleep efficiency, 40–41
sleep functions, 12–25
    body restoration, 15–16
    disease and immune defense, 16–17

emotional tempering and resilience, 21
energy conservation, 21
hormone release, 16
memory storage, 20
waste clearance (glymphatic system), 17–18
sleep hygiene, 81, 137, 138, 144
sleeping pills. *See* sleep medications, prescription
sleep medications, prescription. *See also* medications
daridorexant, 156, 162
doxepin, 163, 164
eszopiclone, 156, 157–158, 159, 164, 268, 293
lemborexant, 156, 162
mechanism of, 158–159
ramelteon, 162, 164
suvorexant, 162, 164
temazepam, 160
trazodone, 162–163, 165
unusual sleep behaviors and, 159
zaleplon, 156, 157, 159, 165, 268
Z-drugs, 156, 157–159, 161, 268
zolpidem, 156, 157, 159, 165, 205, 268, 269–270, 271, 279, 293
sleep needs, 36–37
in adults, 51–52
by age, 43–44, 45
circadian rhythms and, 44, 46–50
measuring and assessing, 37–41
in men vs. women, 52
in older adults, 52
research on, 41–43
sleep efficiency, 40–41
sleep regularity, 41
sleep-wake cycle and, 47–50
in teens, 50–51
time in bed, 37–38
time spent awake, 39–40
time to fall asleep, 38
total sleep time, 40
sleep questionnaires, 114–117
Epworth Sleepiness Scale, 116, 117
Insomnia Severity Index, 114–115
International Restless Legs Severity Scale, 116

Pittsburgh Sleep Quality Index, 116
STOP-Bang, 114
sleep regularity, 41
sleep routine guidelines, 81–95
alcohol and caffeine, 87–88
dinner and nighttime snacks, 86–87
exercise, 89–90
naps, 90–93
nicotine, 88–89
relaxation techniques, 93–95
screens, 89
time and schedules, 83–86
sleep specialists, 122–123
sleep stages, 12–25, 28. *See also* rapid eye movement
N1 (non-REM stage 1), 26, 28
N2 (non-REM stage 2), 27–29
N3 (non-REM stage 3), 28, 29
REM sleep, 28, 29–30
sleep studies (polysomnography), 40, 41, 114, 118–119
actigraphy compared with, 38–39
idiopathic hypersomnia and, 243
for insomnia, 136
narcolepsy and, 230, 238
for narcolepsy and idiopathic hypersomnia, 230, 238–239, 243, 252
for parasomnias, 270, 272, 275, 277
for sleep apnea, 114, 192, 195–199, 204, 212, 213, 224, 228
sleep apnea and, 195, 196
sleep talking, 274, 280
sleep terrors, 112, 268, 272–274, 280
sleep trackers, 38–39. *See also* actigraphy
sleep-wake balance, 131–132
sleep-wake cycle, 23, 47, 156, 232
advanced sleep-wake phase disorder, 285–286, 292
circadian rhythm disorders, 110–111
delayed sleep-wake phase disorder, 285, 292
irregular sleep-wake rhythm disorder, 286–287
non-24-hour sleep-wake rhythm disorder, 286, 293, 301

sleepwalking, 29, 111, 265–266, 267–270, 273
  causes of, 269–270
  diagnosing, 196
  hypnosis for, 280
  as medication side-effect, 268, 269–270, 279
  narcolepsy and, 277
  REM sleep behavior disorder and, 276
  sleep apnea and, 181
slow-wave sleep, 29, 52, 63, 98
smoking. *See* nicotine
social jet lag, 50
somnambulism. *See* sleepwalking
Sonata, 156, 157, 159, 165, 268
spindles, 25, 28
stimulus control therapy, 138–140, 149, 150
stress and worry, 64–65, 94–96, 107, 108
  insomnia and, 124–127, 129–131, 136–137, 145–147
  parasomnias and, 267, 269, 275
  restless legs syndrome and, 254
sudden infant death syndrome (SIDS), 66
suprachiasmatic nucleus, 22, 23, 282–283, 303
suvorexant, 156, 160, 162, 164

T

tasimelteon, 293, 303
tea. *See also* caffeine
  black tea, 88
  caffeine in, 60, 88, 121
  GABA in, 169
teens. *See* adolescence and teens
teeth grinding, 275
temazepam, 160
thalamus, 22, 23
tiagabine, 165
topiramate, 279
trazodone, 162–163, 165, 305
triazolam, 165

tryptophan, 165
type 2 diabetes, 42, 43, 76–77
  insomnia and, 74
  poor sleep and, 76–77
  shift work and, 55, 283
  sleep apnea and, 74, 177, 186, 190
  social jet lag and, 50

V

vaccines, sleep and, 17

W

watch-like sleep trackers, 38, 287. *See also* actigraphy
Wegovy, 209
weighted blankets, 102
weight loss
  bariatric surgery, 224
  obesity hypoventilation syndrome and, 183
  semaglutide, 209
  sleep apnea and, 177, 208, 209–210, 224
  as symptom of AIDS, 229
  as symptom of fatal insomnia, 133
Willis, Thomas, 247
Willis-Ekbom disease, 247. *See also* restless legs syndrome
workplace strategies, 56
worry. *See* stress and worry

Z

zaleplon, 156, 157, 159, 165, 268
Z-drugs, 156, 157–159, 161, 268
  eszopiclone, 156, 157–158, 159, 164, 268, 293
  zaleplon, 156, 157, 159, 165, 268
  zolpidem, 156, 157, 159, 165, 205, 268, 269–270, 271, 279, 293
zeitgebers, 84, 288
zolpidem, 156, 157, 159, 165, 205, 268, 269–270, 271, 279, 293